Speech physiology, speech perception, and acoustic phonetics

In this series:

Speech physiology, speech perception, and acoustic phonetics

Philip Lieberman and Sheila E. Blumstein

Department of Cognitive and Linguistic Sciences, Brown University

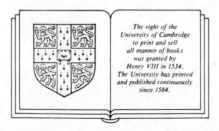

*The right of the
University of Cambridge
to print and sell
all manner of books
was granted by
Henry VIII in 1534.
The University has printed
and published continuously
since 1584.*

Cambridge University Press

Cambridge

New York   Port Chester   Melbourne   Sydney

Published by the Press Syndicate of the University of Cambridge
The Pitt Building, Trumpington Street, Cambridge CB2 1RP
40 West 20th Street, New York, NY 10011, USA
10 Stamford Road, Oakleigh, Melbourne 3166, Australia

First published 1988
Reprinted 1990

Printed in Great Britain by The Bath Press, Avon

British Library cataloguing in publication data
Lieberman, Philip
    Speech physiology, speech perception, and
    acoustic phonetics. – (Cambridge studies in
    speech science and communication).
    1. Speech
    I. Title   II. Blumstein, Sheila
    612'.78   QP306

Library of Congress cataloguing in publication data
Lieberman, Philip.
    Speech physiology, speech perception, and acoustic phonetics.
    (Cambridge studies in speech science and communication)
    Bibliography.
    Includes index.
    1. Speech – Physiological aspects.   2. Speech
perception.   3. Phonetics, Acoustic.   I. Blumstein,
Sheila.   II. Title.   III. Series.
QP306.L53   1988   612'.78   87–13187

ISBN 0 521 30866 6 hard covers
ISBN 0 521 31357 0 paperback

To our parents

Contents

Contents

Figures

List of figures

List of figures

Preface

The study of speech is relevant to a variety of different fields such as psychology, linguistics, anthropology, primatology, electrical engineering, and computer science, as well as the fields of speech science and language pathology. In teaching introductory courses on the production and perception of speech, and on the procedures of acoustic phonetics and speech physiology, we have encountered students with very different academic backgrounds. Some of these students have had a working knowledge of the acoustics of speech, electrical circuit theory, experimental psychology, or the anatomy of the vocal tract. Many of our students, however, have had very little quantitative knowledge of physics, anatomy, or psychology. Others may be familiar with one area but are deficient in other aspects of the study of speech. We have felt for some time that there is a need for a text that guides students from different backgrounds to a quantitative understanding of speech without their having to take a two or three year sequence of specialized courses. This book thus provides a step-by-step introduction that starts with simple examples that put the subject into perspective. It ends with a detailed exposition of recent theories and data. The book assumes no knowledge of physics or mathematics beyond the high school level. The background that is necessary for understanding the physics of sound, the source-filter theory of speech production, and the principles that underlie electrical and computer models of speech production is presented in stages and is illustrated by means of simple examples. Problem sets are presented at the end of each chapter. These problems test the concepts that we think are basic to the topics discussed in each chapter. Other, more complex questions undoubtedly will suggest themselves to the more advanced student since we will discuss issues that are, as yet, unresolved.

The reader should be able to follow the results of primary research papers that are presented and understand the implications of these results for his or her own area of special interest, whether that is speech therapy, phonological theory, psycholinguistics, neurolinguistics, anthropology, etc. The implications of quantitative studies involving techniques like cineradiography, sound spectrography, dichotic listening, electromyography, computer modeling, etc., are often unintelligible to the nonspecialist; this book should make these results accessible by providing a knowledge of relevant theories and techniques and also of the deficiencies of these theories and techniques. We have tried to convey some of the problems and some of the exhilaration that one encounters in doing research. Science is not the cut-and-dried gathering of "facts" that it sometimes seems to be in textbooks where theories are supported by armies of "facts" and "proofs" organized in divisions and battalions. Every theory has its deficiencies, and the "art" of science is in deciding which theories are most promising and how they may be tested. The chapter on the analysis of speech (Chapter 5) which notes the basic techniques of tape recording, as well as the use of the sound spectrograph and computer analysis, can serve as the basis of a course in experimental phonetics. The chapters on speech production (Chapter 6), speech perception (Chapter 7), and phonetic theory (Chapter 8) present various experimental techniques and unresolved questions. The chapter on the development of speech in children and its "dissolution" in aphasia (Chapter 9) shows how these experimental techniques can be applied to address basic research issues in the biology and neurology of speech. The text thus highlights problems that students can investigate. A number of original studies have been completed and published by undergraduate and graduate students using this text. Most of these students had no technical background before they started. The reader obviously can and should supplement this material with primary research papers as he or she becomes more familiar with the field. Detailed charts and illustrations that can serve as reference material, as well as pedagogic aids, are therefore provided through-out the book, as well as references to primary research papers. Chapter 10 presents a discussion of some of the known acoustic correlates to the sounds of speech. The book may thus be useful as a convenient reference source. Our basic aim, however, in writing this book has been to make more people aware of a very new and exciting field, and to start them working in it.

Acknowledgements

We would like to acknowledge fruitful discussions that we have had over the course of many years with Roman Jakobson, Kenneth N. Stevens, Alvin Liberman, Franklin S. Cooper, and Peter Ladefoged. The friendship and support of these colleagues have helped us shape our own views of the nature of speech. The advance of science is inextricably linked to the development of analytical techniques; in this connection, we would like to acknowledge the extraordinary contributions of John Mertus who developed the BLISS system for the analysis of speech and the implementation of psychoacoustic experiments. John has been a valued colleague in our research. To John Gilbert who read through our first draft and made invaluable suggestions we give our thanks. We would also like to gratefully acknowledge Patricia Rigby's dedicated efforts at decoding illegible copy and taming recalcitrant word processors, and Harry Mourachian's artistic talents in helping create graphs and figures. To our students, we would like to express our thanks for their helpful comments, vigorous debates, and insightful questions – Shari Baum, Susan Behrens, Martha Burton, Carol Chapin, William E. Cooper, Allard Jongman, William Katz, Patricia Keating, Cathy Kubaska, Kathleen Kurowski, Aditi Lahiri, Karen Landahl, Molly Mack, Joan Sereno, Philip Shinn, Vicki Tartter, and Chiu Yu Tseng. Finally, to the editorial staff at Cambridge University Press and particularly to Penny Carter and Sue Glover, we gratefully acknowledge their dedication, patience, and professionalism in seeing this manuscript through to its final publication. This work was supported in part by Grant NS 15123 to Brown University.

1

Introduction

The study of language and the sounds of speech can be traced back at least to the Greek and Sanskrit grammarians of the third and fourth centuries BC. The explicit study of speech science began in the eighteenth century when Ferrein (1741) attempted to explain how the vocal cords produced phonation. Ferrein's studies were not an isolated event. Kratzenstein (1780) and von Kempelen (1791) attempted to explain how the vowels and consonants of human speech were produced by synthesizing sounds using artificial "talking machines." There indeed may have been earlier attempts at constructing talking machines; La Mettrie (1747) discusses some of these early attempts, but we lack detailed records. By the mid nineteenth century Müller (1848) had formulated the source–filter theory of speech production, which is consistent with the most recent data and still guides research on human speech as well as the vocal communications of other animals. Although Müller's theory was further developed later in the nineteenth century, particularly by Hermann (1894), the modern period of speech science is really quite recent, dating back to the late 1930s, where devices like the sound spectrograph, and techniques like high-speed photography, cineradiography, and electromyography made new data available. Quantitative studies like those of Chiba and Kajiyama (1941), Joos (1948), Peterson and Barney (1952), Stevens and House (1955), and Fant (1960) refined and tested the traditional phonetic theories of the nineteenth century and provided the framework for comprehensive, biologically-oriented studies of speech production, speech perception, and phonetics. The advent and general availability of digital computers made quantitative modeling studies possible. New techniques for speech synthesis and psychoacoustic experiments have made it possible to explore the fundamental properties of human speech.

We are beginning to understand how human speech is produced, how it is perceived, and how the physiological properties of the vocal tract and the neural mechanisms of the brain contribute to speech processing. We also are beginning to understand how human language and human speech evolved and how other animals communicate. The development of speech and language in infants and children is being explored, and new possibilities are opening for the diagnosis and amelioration of various speech pathologies.

The focus of this introduction to speech physiology and acoustic phonetics is thus to provide a background to the "new" speech science. An understanding of the acoustics of speech, the physiology of speech production, and the special factors that are involved in the perception of speech is a prerequisite for further study of the pathologies of speech production or the neurological impairment of either speech production or speech perception. It is also necessary for the development of quantitative, predictive phonetic and phonological studies. While linguists have studied the sound structure of language, exploring the processes of sound change and the structure of sound systems in language, it is the study of speech science which may provide the explanations for *why* sounds change in the way they do and *why* the sound systems of natural language are structured in the way that they are. This introduction is no substitute for a traditional phonetics text, focused on teaching people how to make transcriptions of various languages and dialects. The training techniques that phoneticians use are not included in this book because our objective is to understand the biological mechanisms that are the basis not only of human speech, but also of vocal communication in many other animals.

Readers who have a good background in high-school mathematics should have little difficulty in following the discussions of the acoustics of speech production or the source–filter theory of speech production. Readers who have a more advanced background may be able to skim appropriate chapters.

Although readers may find this book a useful reference source, its primary function is pedagogic. It should be viewed as an introduction to the physiology of speech and acoustic phonetics. Many current problems are not discussed in detail, and the advanced reader may be familiar with topics that have been omitted. Everyone, however, should encounter new material and indeed should note that speech science is still a frontier with many gaps in our knowledge yet to be filled. It is becoming apparent that human speech is an integral part of human linguistic ability. The biological bases of human speech are complex and appear to follow from the Darwinian process of natural selection acting over at least 250 000 years to yield specialized anatomical and neural mechanisms in *Homo sapiens* (Lieberman, 1984). The gaps in our knowledge concerning the biological bases of human speech thus reflect the difficulties inherent in understanding the nature of language and human cognition of which speech forms a crucial part.

A qualitative introduction to the physiology of speech

Physiology is the science that deals with the function of biological systems. An anatomist, for example, could describe the bones and muscles of the human foot without considering how these elements work together in activities like bipedal locomotion. A physiologist would have to consider these same bones and muscles in terms of their functional value in locomotion and other activities. In fact, anatomists usually take account of the function of the bones, muscle, and soft tissue that they describe since the physiological or functional approach is inherently more integrated than a strictly anatomical one. The physiological method of describing the anatomy of human speech production indicates what elements have a functional value with regard to speech production and what anatomical elements are irrelevant. We thus do not have to catalogue every bone and variation in the soft tissue of the mouth, pharynx, and nose. We can focus on the elements that have a functional role in the production of speech. So instead of listing every bone, cartilage, and muscle, we will start with a broad outline of the physiology of speech and relevant anatomical structures. We will add more detail in later chapters when we consider specific aspects of the physiology of speech production.

The three physiological components of speech production

It is convenient and functionally appropriate to consider speech production in terms of three components. The larynx has come to be used as the reference point for this three-way split. The larynx is a complex structure which we will discuss in the pages that follow. You can feel the thyroid cartilage of your larynx if you put your hand against your throat while you swallow. The *vocal cords* are the laryngeal anatomical structures which rapidly open and close during the process of *phonation*. The term *glottal* refers to the opening between the vocal cords of the larynx. The three major physiologic components of speech production are usually described with reference to the glottis. In Figure 2.1 the three components are sketched.

   (1) Below the larynx, we have the *subglottal* component which consists of the lungs and associated respiratory musculature. The subglottal system is

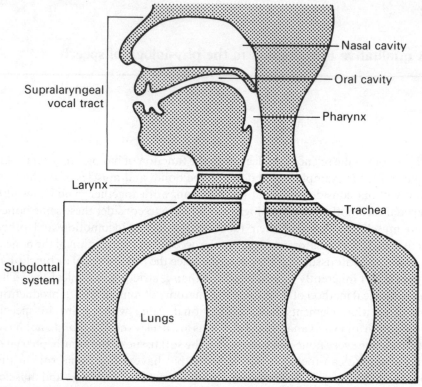

Figure 2.1. The three physiologic components of human speech production.

sketched in Figure 2.1 as it might be seen in an idealized frontal X-ray view. The *trachea* or windpipe leads down from the larynx and bifurcates into two airways that each lead into a lung. The subglottal component generates the air flow that powers speech production

(2) The larynx is also sketched in Figure 2.1 as a sort of X-ray frontal view. We will use more realistic sketches and photographs when we discuss the anatomy, control, and activity of the larynx in more detail. The primary role of the larynx in the production of speech is to convert a relatively steady flow of air out from the lungs into a series of almost periodic, i.e. *"quasi-periodic,"* puffs of air. The larynx does this by rapidly closing and opening the airway by moving the vocal cords together or pulling them apart. As the vocal cords move inwards and outwards the glottal opening closes or opens. A puff of air occurs each time the larynx briefly opens up. (The relationship between air flow and the glottal opening is similar to what happens when you open and close the water valve of your sink; the water flow increases as you open the valve and decreases as you close the valve.) The puffs of air contain acoustic

energy at audible frequencies. The larynx thus is a valve that can rapidly open and close, generating a *"source"* of acoustic energy.

(3) In Figure 2.1 we have sketched the *supralaryngeal vocal tract* above the larynx. The supralaryngeal vocal tract consists of the airways of the nose, mouth and pharynx. It is shown here as a lateral (side) view. During the production of speech, the supralaryngeal airway acts as a variable acoustic *filter* that acts on the source of acoustic energy. It is a variable acoustic filter because the speaker changes the *shape* of his vocal tract as he speaks. The supralaryngeal vocal tract lets proportionately more acoustic energy through it at certain frequencies that are called *formant frequencies.*

It is important to note at this point that these three components, the subglottal system, larynx, and supralaryngeal vocal tract, all perform functions necessary to maintain life, quite apart from their activity relative to speech production. These primary vegetative, or life-supporting, functions have crucially affected the anatomical "design" of the tongue, larynx, nose, lungs, etc., and the physiology of respiration, chewing, swallowing, lung protection, etc. Over millions of years there has been natural selection for mutations that facilitate these functions (Darwin, 1859; Negus, 1949). Many of the characteristics of the anatomical mechanisms that we use to produce human speech reflect these adaptations. Human speech is thus, in part, structured by the constraints of physiological mechanisms whose primary purpose is nonlinguistic.

Some of the characteristics of the larynx do appear to reflect adaptations that enhance communication in humans and other animals (Negus, 1949). There are also certain characteristics of the human supralaryngeal vocal tract that presently appear only in *Homo sapiens* (Lieberman, 1975, 1984). Together, these various physiological constraints exert a strong force on the particular form that human speech has taken. In this chapter we will discuss these three components in a simplified manner in order to keep the total process of speech production in mind as we go into more detail in later chapters.

The subglottal respiratory system

The lungs and associated musculature often are not discussed with regard to their activity during the production of speech. Their activity during the production of speech is, however, very interesting because it derives from the general vegetative functions of the respiratory system without being completely similar. In other words, speech production for the most part is inherently structured in terms of the "normal," nonspeech characteristics of the lungs and respiratory muscles, but there are some additional factors that

5

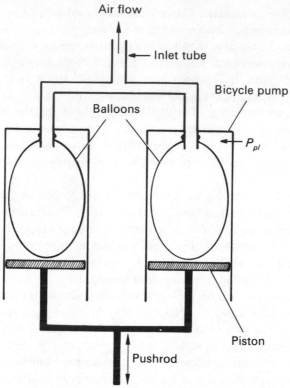

Figure 2.2. A mechanical model of the subglottal respiratory system.

appear to enter into the production of speech and activities like singing. The best way to approach the discussion of the subglottal respiratory system is to describe in simple terms how the lungs work. The respiratory system is put together in a manner that is not immediately obvious. Stetson (1951), for example, proposed a theory that attempted to explain the linguistic and physiological bases of the syllable as a unit of speech. Stetson's theory is unfortunately flawed because he misinterpreted the function of the lungs during quiet respiration and speech.

In Figure 2.2 we have sketched a simple model of the subglottal respiratory system. The model consists of two bicycle pumps that have their pushrods rigidly linked together. A crossbar and handle have been welded to the two pushrods. Each pump contains a large rubber balloon attached to the inlet tube. The two inlet tubes are linked together and merge into a single tube. This single tube is analogous to the trachea of the human respiratory system. The air entering the two bicycle pumps flows through this inlet tube into the inlet tubes of the two bicycle pumps, where it goes into the balloons. This mechanical model isolates some of the physiological aspects of the subglottal system that are of interest for speech production. The linked bicycle pump rods in Figure 2.2 are rigidly connected to the pushrod. If the pushrod moves upwards, it will move the two pistons upwards, reducing the volume inside each bicycle pump. If the pushrod moves downwards, the pistons will also move downwards, increasing the volume inside each bicycle pump.

A general principle of physics tells us that the air pressure multiplied by the volume of an enclosed container must equal a constant value. The space between the inside of each pump and the outside of the balloon is an enclosed volume. This space is analogous to the *pleural space* of the lung. Your lungs are not rigidly attached to your rib cage; there is an enclosed volume, the pleural space, between the lung and chest wall. The internal volume of the balloons is analogous to the internal volume of the lungs. In the equation below P_{pl} represents the air pressure within this pleural space and V represents its volume.

$$P_{pl}(V) = C$$

where

P_{pl} = the air pressure of the "pleural" space between the inside of the pump body and balloon

V = "pleural" volume; the space between the inside of the pump body and balloon

C = a constant value

The "pleural" air pressure within each pump body (the air pressure in the space between the inside of the pump and the balloon) will therefore fall as the pushrod moves downwards, increasing the volume inside each bicycle pump. The air pressure will obviously be less than it was at the instant of time before the pushrod moved downwards. The outside air pressure is manifested on the inside of each balloon because the balloon is connected through the inlet tubes to the outside. The balloons therefore will expand as outside air enters. In other words, the two balloons will stretch and expand, storing more air as the pushrod is pulled down.

Note that it takes more energy to suck a given volume of air into this system than into a simple bicycle pump that did not have a balloon placed over its inlet tube. When you blow up a rubber balloon you have to stretch the rubber walls of the balloon. The rubber walls of the balloon are elastic and they store up energy as they expand. You therefore have to provide the energy that is stored in the stretched, elastic balloon walls. This stored elastic energy is, of course, released if you release a rubber balloon after you have blown it up. The *elastic recoil* force of the balloon walls will force the air out of the balloon under

7

pressure. Everyone has probably played with a flying balloon. You blow it up and then release it; the power for flight comes from the energy that was stored in the balloon.

What will happen in our model of the subglottal respiratory system if we release the pushrod with the balloons in their expanded state, i.e. after the pushrod has been pulled down as far as it will go? The balloons obviously will collapse and air will flow out of the "tracheal" tube. The elastic recoil force of the balloons will force air out and the pushrods will move inwards, following the collapsing balloons. It takes muscular force to get air into this model when you pull the rod out during inspiration. In contrast, during expiration air will go out of the system without your applying any force. You could force the air out faster during expiration if you also pushed the rod inwards, but you do not have to. The energy stored in the elastic balloons can provide the force that pushes the air out during expiration.

This model holds for the subglottal respiratory systems of virtually all air-breathing higher animals. The internal volume of the bicycle pump that is not taken up by the balloon is called the *pleural cavity* (or *pleural space*). Most of the energy that we expend to transfer air into and out of our lungs comes from the inspiratory muscles that expand the pleural space. As the pleural space increases its volume, the volume of the elastic lung-balloon increases. Energy is stored in the elastic expansion of each lung. During expiration the elastic recoil of the lungs furnishes much of the energy that is necessary to push air out of the lungs through the larynx and supralaryngeal air passages. The balance of force provided by the elastic recoil and various inspiratory and expiratory muscles is variable during the production of human speech and is an example of how the physiological constraints that underlie the production of human speech ultimately structure the form of human speech. Other variable forces also act during the respiratory cycle. The force of gravity, for example, acts differently when a person stands up or lies down. The control problem is actually quite complex. We will return to the topic of the control of the subglottal respiratory system after we discuss the necessary background material in the chapters that follow; for the moment we will continue our preliminary discussion of the respiratory system.

In Figure 2.3 some of the muscles that are active in the regulation of respiration are sketched. This view is more realistic than our first two diagrams. We have several different inspiratory muscles. The *intercostal* muscles, for example, which are interwoven with the ribs, can act to increase the pleural space by expanding the rib cage. The *external intercostals*, which are closer to the outside surface of the body, and most of the *internal intercostal* muscles are inspiratory muscles. Figure 2.3 does not show the *diaphragm*, which is a muscle that can move downwards to expand the pleural space.

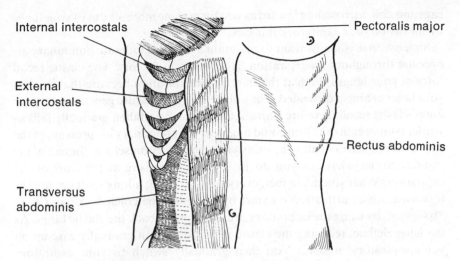

Internal intercostals

External intercostals

Transversus abdominis

Pectoralis major

Rectus abdominis

Figure 2.3. Some of the muscles that control respiration.

Though the diaphragm is active during quiet respiration, it does not appear to be used when people speak, sing, or play musical instruments that require precise regulation of pulmonary air pressure (Bouhuys, 1974). Part of the internal intercostals and the *abdominal* muscles can act to force air out of the lungs. They thus can act as expiratory muscles. These muscles are all used to maintain a steady pulmonary air pressure while we speak or sing. The term *pulmonary* here refers to the lungs. The pulmonary air pressure, hence, is the air pressure inside the lungs. The control pattern of the respiratory muscles that maintains a steady pulmonary air pressure while the lungs collapse during expiration is fairly complex. If we return to our simple balloon model the problem becomes evident. Consider the results of the following simple experiment that you can perform yourself. Blow up a balloon. When the balloon is full, release it. What happens? The balloon flies around. At the start it goes fairly fast, but it rapidly slows down and finally falls to the floor. The balloon is flying fast at first because the pressure of the air inside it is highest when the balloon is distended. As the balloon collapses, the air pressure falls and the balloon flies slower and slower. If you now perform some simple exercises you can sense the pulmonary control problems.

Start by taking a deep breath, i.e. a large inspiration. Put your hand a few inches in front of your open mouth and let your breath out while you relax. You will note that the air streaming out of your mouth has less force towards the end of the breath. This reflects the gradual release of the elastic recoil force of your lungs. Repeat the procedure a second time, wait until your breath ceases, and then push some more air out. You should be able to sense your rib cage and abdomen pulling inward as you force some more air out of your lungs by means of your expiratory muscles.

Suppose that you now want to maintain a steady, moderate pulmonary air pressure throughout an expiration. How can you do this? The elastic recoil force of your lungs is high at the start of the expiration because that is when your lungs are most distended. The pulmonary air pressure generated by your lungs' elastic recoil therefore starts at a high value and then gradually falls as you let your breath out. You could augment the pulmonary air pressure at the end of the relaxed expiration by using your expiratory muscles at the end of the expiration, but what can you do to lower the pressure at the *start* of the expiration? What you do, in fact, every time you utter a long sentence are the following muscular feats. You start by opposing the collapse of your lung "balloons" by using the inspiratory muscles to hold back the elastic lungs. As the lungs deflate, reducing the elastic recoil force, you gradually ease up on your inspiratory muscles. You then gradually switch to your expiratory muscles, maintaining an even pulmonary air pressure throughout the operation. Recent studies on the "programming" of the respiratory muscles during speech, which we will discuss in Chapter 6, indicate that speakers are unconsciously aware of these problems and that they unconsciously organize the control of their respiratory muscles in terms of the length of a sentence before they utter a sound.

The biological mechanisms that underlie respiration obviously include *neural control devices*. The primary function of the respiratory system is to provide oxygen. Human beings have a system of chemoreceptors that monitor the levels of dissolved carbon dioxide and oxygen in our blood and cerebrospinal fluid (Bouhuys, 1974). These chemoreceptors during quiet respiration initiate respiration when the level of carbon dioxide rises too high and conversely slow respiration when the oxygen level climbs. The chemoreceptor systems can operate rapidly; when you are in a small room breathing stale air, a single breath of pure oxygen will lead to a temporary reduction of ventilation (Dejours, 1963). When we talk, we override these chemoreceptor systems. The air flow requirements for speech production do not always match those necessary for basic, vegetative life-support, and the demands of speech usually prevail. At low levels of physical activity, people thus take in more air when they talk than they need to for supporting life. We will return, in Chapter 6, to these aspects of the control of speech production which appear to reflect evolution for communication.

The larynx

The larynx is a device that transforms what would, in its absence, be a steady flow of air from the lungs into a series of puffs of air. The larynx is present in all terrestrial animals and derives from the valve that protected the lungs of primitive lungfish. Although it evolved from a device whose primary function was the protection of the lungs, the larynx is also adapted for phonation (Negus, 1949). The periodic series of puffs of air constitute the source of acoustic energy that characterizes *phonation*. The vocal calls of many air-breathing animals, even simple ones like frogs (Stuart, 1958; Lieberman, 1984), involve phonation. Sounds like the English vowels /a/ and /i/ usually are phonated, as are sounds like the English consonants /m/ and /v/. These sounds occur in the words *mama* /mama/, *meat* /mit/, and *veal* /vil/. The croak of a bullfrog is phonated, as is a sheep's bleat.

In Figure 2.4 a set of frames from a high-speed movie of the human larynx is presented. The photographs show the vocal cords, often called *folds*, gradually adducting or moving together. The vocal cords consist of muscles and ligaments on a cartilaginous support, all of which are covered by a membrane. Cartilage is a material that generally is rigid or semirigid. The vocal cords are complex structures that do not really resemble cords. The term *cords* was first used by the eighteenth-century French scientist Ferrein (1741), who published one of the first theories that attempted to account for how phonation occurred. Ferrein thought that the vocal cords acted like the strings of a violin or a harp. His theory was not correct but his terminology, in so far as it has a functional derivation, is perhaps somewhat better than the term "vocal folds" which is often used to describe these complex structures. The term "folds" better describes how these structures look when they are examined by looking down someone's open mouth using a laryngeal mirror. However, it does not really describe their complex internal structure, nor does it suggest their unique physiological function which is quite different from that of any other "fold" of tissue. We shall therefore use the term *vocal cords* since it has historical precedent and follows from a physiological assessment of how phonation occurs.

The opening between the vocal cords is called the *glottis*. Terms like "subglottal air pressure" therefore refer to the air pressure immediately below the glottal opening.

The first frame in Figure 2.4 shows the vocal cords at the moment when they began to adduct. The second photographic frame shows the same speaker's larynx about 50 milliseconds later. (A millisecond (msec) is one-thousandth of a second; it is a convenient unit of time for describing the events that occur during the production and perception of speech.) The third frame shows his vocal cords fully adducted at the start of phonation. Note that it took about 100 milliseconds for this speaker's vocal cords to close before he could start phonation. The muscles of the larynx actively close the larynx, and tense the vocal cords before and during the act of phonation. They do not, however, furnish the power for phonation. That power comes from the air stream

11

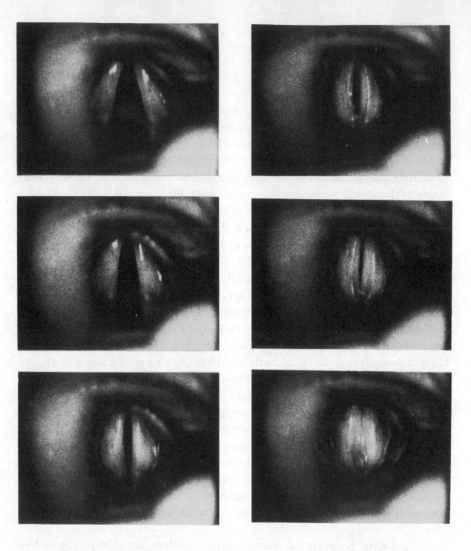

Figure 2.4 (left). Three frames from a high-speed movie showing the vocal cords gradually moving together before the start of phonation. A Fastax high-speed camera exposed these frames at a rate of 10 000 pictures per second (Lieberman, 1963). The posterior part of the vocal cords is oriented towards the bottom of each frame. The uppermost picture shows the vocal cords open wide for inspiration. The middle frame was exposed about 50 milliseconds later. It shows the vocal cords partially closed. The bottom frame was exposed 50 milliseconds later. It shows the vocal cords closed just before phonation started and before the vocal folds are fully closed.

Figure 2.5 (right). Three frames from the same high-speed movie as Figure 2.4, exposed during phonation. The top frame shows the maximum opening during one cycle of phonation. The bottom frame, exposed 7 milliseconds later, shows the vocal cords closed completely.

passing out from the lungs. The process of phonation involves an alternation of forces. The air flow out of the lungs first pushes the vocal cords apart, letting lots of air through. The vocal cords are then pulled together by the elastic properties of their stretched tissue and the suction generated by the flow of air through the glottal constriction. The force generated by the air flow through the glottal constriction, the *Bernoulli force*, is similar to the suction that occurs when a bus passes close to a car at a high speed.

The pictures in Figure 2.5 show three frames from the same high-speed movie, but they show the vocal cords during phonation. Note that the change in opening is not as great as in Figure 2.4 and that it occurs within 7 milliseconds, i.e. far more quickly. Phonation consists of the vocal cords rapidly opening and closing under the *control* of the laryngeal muscles, *powered* by the air flow from the lungs. The respiratory muscles can also exert control on phonation; we will go into the details later.

If you purse your lips and blow through them to imitate the sound that a horse makes, you can simulate the process of phonation. The force of air going out of your mouth furnishes the power that produces the sound. The sound comes from the acoustic energy generated by your lips interrupting the flow of air out of your mouth.

The supralaryngeal vocal tract

Like the role of the larynx, the role of the supralaryngeal vocal tract in speech production was known in the eighteenth century. In 1779 Kratzenstein constructed a set of tubes that he supposed were similar to the shape of the human vocal tract during the production of the vowels of Russian. The Academy of Sciences of St Petersburg, Russia, had offered its annual prize for explaining the physiological differences between the five vowels that occur in Russian. Kratzenstein (1780) used these tubes to filter the output of vibrating reeds and thereby "explained" the physiological differences that differentiated these vowels. In 1791 von Kempelen demonstrated his speech-synthesizing machine. The relationship between the sounds of speech and the supralaryngeal vocal tract is, in part, analogous to that between the pipes of an organ and musical notes. In a pipe organ, the length and shape of each pipe (whether the pipe is open at both ends or closed at one end) determines the musical quality of the note produced by that pipe. The organ pipes act as acoustic filters that are interposed between the common source of sound, which can excite any particular pipe, and the listener's ear. When we play a pipe organ, we connect different pipes to the source. The production of human speech involves changing the shape and length of a "plastic" pipe, the airways of the human supralaryngeal vocal tract. It would in principle be possible to make a pipe organ that had a single plastic pipe whose shape was distended or contracted through the action of electrically controlled motors. Such a pipe organ would be a closer mechanical analog to the human supralaryngeal vocal tract.

We can also construct electrical and computer-implemented analogs to the human supralaryngeal vocal tract. These analogs, which are the descendants of Kratzenstein's and von Kempelen's eighteenth-century models, have yielded important insights on the nature of human speech and the vocal communications of many other animals. We will return to this topic.

The neural processing of speech

Before we go on to introduce some of the physical and mathematical concepts that are necessary to explore the production and perception of speech in more detail, we should point out the match that exists between the production and the perception of sound. Frogs are among the simplest animals that produce calls by means of a laryngeal source. We never hear the laryngeal source directly because the frogs' supralaryngeal airways, like those of a human being, act as a filter. Electrophysiological and behavioral experiments (Frishkopf and Goldstein, 1963; Capranica, 1965), which we will discuss in greater detail in Chapter 7, demonstrate that bullfrogs have "devices" in their auditory systems that are tuned to respond selectively to their mating calls. The acoustic characteristics of the mating calls are fully specified by the physiology of the frogs' larynges and supralaryngeal vocal tracts. Frogs thus have auditory systems that have, in part, been designed to respond to the vocal calls that frogs make.

Similar though more complex neural devices adapted to the perception of speech appear to exist in human beings. Since the late nineteenth century, it has been evident that certain parts of the human brain appear to be especially involved with the production of human speech (Broca, 1861) and the processing of language (Wernicke, 1874). The research of the past thirty years has shown that both the production and perception of human speech involve specialized neural devices. Human beings also have a supralaryngeal vocal tract that differs from those of other living nonhuman primates as well as the reconstructed vocal tracts of extinct hominids. The human supralaryngeal vocal tract and the neural devices that are necessary for the production and perception of human speech appear to be "matched" to yield a functional system (Lieberman, 1975, 1984). We will return to these topics in the chapters that follow.

Exercises

1. Why does human speech typically take place during the expiratory phase of respiration? Consider the role of the inspiratory muscles and the elastic recoil of the lungs.

2. One of the consequences of the pathologic condition of emphysema is the loss of elasticity of the lungs. What effect do you think this pathology would have on the production of speech?

3. How would the speech of a speaker of English whose larynx was surgically removed because of cancer of the larynx differ from that of a normal speaker?

4. Suppose that you were able to position a microphone directly above a speaker's vocal cords so that you could listen to their acoustic output. Would the speaker's speech be more or less intelligible than it would be if you positioned the microphone at the speaker's lips? Explain the basis for your answer.

3

Basic acoustics

The principles that underlie the processes of speech production and speech perception are difficult to discuss without making use of the physical concepts of wave motion, periodicity, frequency, and amplitude. These concepts are, fortunately, fairly simple and straightforward. We will also discuss the use and the physical meaning of graphs as they relate to the description of physical measurements, and conclude with an elementary description of the frequency analysis of acoustic signals and the properties of filters. Readers who have appropriate backgrounds in the physical sciences, mathematics, or engineering will undoubtedly find this chapter superfluous because we will introduce and explain these concepts by means of simple everyday examples, using a minimum of mathematical formalism. The examples that we start with – the measurement of temperature, ocean waves, and so on – have nothing to do with the acoustics of speech, but they illustrate in a direct manner the physical concepts that we want to develop.

Graphs and physical measurements

Let us start by considering the topic of graphs and their interpretation. Suppose that you were asked to read the temperature at four-hour intervals from a thermometer mounted in the shade on the back of your house. You could record the temperature that you read at each four-hour interval in the form of a list. The list, for example, might look like that in Table 3.1 for the three-day period August 7 to August 9. An equivalent way of recording this temperature information would be to make a graph. The graph of Figure 3.1 is equivalent to Table 3.1.

The graph is organized as follows. The vertical scale records the temperature registered on the thermometer. The horizontal scale records the time at which the reading was made. The first observation of temperature of the graph of Figure 3.1 therefore must be interpreted as indicating a temperature of 80 degrees Fahrenheit (°F) at 9 a.m. The observation is marked by means of the black dot that lines up with 80 degrees on the vertical scale of the graph and with 9 a.m., August 7, on the horizontal scale. This fact is, of course, recorded

Table 3.1. *List of temperatures recorded at four-hour intervals for three days*

Temperature (°F)	Time
80	9 a.m. August 7
90	1 p.m.
95	5 p.m.
80	9 p.m.
70	1 a.m. August 8
60	5 a.m.
82	9 a.m.
88	1 p.m.
94	5 p.m.
75	9 p.m.
60	1 a.m. August 9
55	5 a.m.
80	9 a.m.

in Table 3.1, which also indicates that the temperature at 9 a.m. on August 7 was 80 degrees. The next black dot on the graph indicates that the temperature was 90 degrees at 1 p.m. This fact is again indicated by the information in Table 3.1. The graph thus loses none of the information recorded in Table 3.1. If the graph did no more than display the information recorded in Table 3.1 in a different manner, there would be little point in bothering to make the graph. The graph, however, does much more. It allows us to derive from the temperature readings interpretations that are not as apparent when we view the data in Table 3.1.

The first interpretation of the data in Table 3.1, implicit in the graph, is that the temperature changed gradually and in the same direction between temperature observations. The black dots that mark the actual temperature readings recorded are connected by a line, and we could estimate that the temperature at 10 a.m. on August 7, for example, was probably 82 degrees. Note that we did not really read the temperature at 10 a.m. We have derived this estimate of the temperature from the graph. We could have made the same estimate from the data of Table 3.1, but it is more apparent in the graph. The graph directly presents this "interpolation" between the actual temperature readings taken at 9 a.m. and at 1 p.m.

The interpolation is based on our knowledge of how temperature changes occur. We know, for example, that the temperature normally does not abruptly rise 100 degrees and then fall 100 degrees in ten minutes. We also know that there has to be some value of temperature at all times. This real-world knowledge is built into this particular graph in which continuous lines

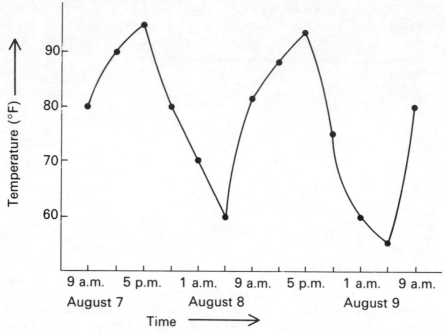

Figure 3.1. Graph of temperatures plotted from data in Table 3.1.

connect the data points. It is important to consider the nature of the data that one is plotting in a graph since these conditions are not always met.

Waveforms and periodicity

The visual pattern of this graph where we have plotted temperature as a *function of time* also throws into relief other interpretations of the temperature observations. The term *function of time* implies that there is a dependency between the temperature readings and time. This is obviously true since the temperature readings were taken at four-hour intervals. It is also true in a deeper sense since there is an overall relationship or pattern between the temperature readings and the time of day. This is apparent from the shape, that is, the "form" of the graph of Figure 3.1. The temperature goes up to a peak value at 5 p.m. each day and then descends to a minimum value at about 5 a.m. the next day. The temperature readings are not identical for the same hour of each day, but the pattern is quite similar. We can see from the graph that the temperature pattern over this interval of three days is *quasi-periodic*, or almost periodic. A *periodic event* is one that repeats itself. The *periodicity* or *period* of the temperature cycle is 24 hours. In other words, the temperature variations

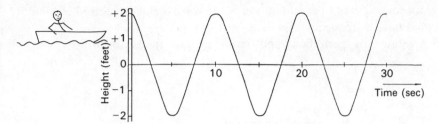

Figure 3.2. Graph of water height showing the 10 second period of the waveform.

tend to repeat themselves every 24 hours. It is obvious to everyone that the temperature variations are periodic, with a period of 24 hours, because the sun rises and sets each day. We do not need a graph to tell us this. However, the graph shows the periodicity in an obvious manner. The periodicity of the temperature variations tends to be buried in the data of Table 3.1.

Frequency

We can make graphs that present virtually any measurement. Graphs allow us to readily "see" periodic relationships. We could, for example, record the height of the water as it was measured against a ruler nailed to the side of one of the posts supporting the end of a pier at the Atlantic City beach. We could, in principle, record the height of the water every second and plot it, that is, record it on a graph.

The sketch in Figure 3.2 shows a person in a boat observing the height of the water against this ruler. The 0-line of this ruler represents the height of the water if it was absolutely quiet, e.g. no waves at all. The person reads the height of the water, which has waves every 10 seconds on this day, and plots it on the graph to the right. The vertical scale, the *ordinate*, is the height of the water. The horizontal scale, the *abscissa*, is time. Note that the height of the water (± 2 feet) *at this fixed point in space – the end of the pier –* is plotted as a function of time. The period of the *waveform* refers to the shape of the plotted data on the graph. The period is 10 seconds (sec), because the waveform repeats itself every 10 seconds. A complete cycle from maximum to minimum and back to maximum occurs every 10 seconds. In 1 minute (min) the waveform would repeat itself six times.

If we wanted to note how often this waveform repeated itself, we could say that it had a period of 10 seconds, or we could say that it repeated itself with a frequency of 6 cycles per minute. The term *frequency* thus refers to the number of times that a periodic event repeats itself for some standard interval of time. An ocean wave that had a period of 30 seconds, that is ½ minute, would have a frequency of 2 cycles per minute. An ocean wave that had a period of $\frac{1}{4}$ minute would have a frequency of 4 cycles per minute.

Algebraically, periodicity and frequency have the relationship

$$f = \frac{1}{T}$$

where f = frequency
and T = the duration of the period
An event that had a period of $\frac{1}{50}$ second would have a frequency of 50 cycles per second, because

$$f = \frac{1}{T} = \frac{1}{\frac{1}{50}} = 50$$

An event that had a period of 0.01 second ($\frac{1}{100}$ second in decimal notation) would have a frequency of 100 cycles per second. We will encounter the term *Hertz* (abbreviated Hz) as a measure of frequency when we discuss sound waves. A frequency of 1 Hz is, by definition, equal to 1 cycle per second, 50 Hz to 50 cycles per second, etc.

Sinusoidal waves

Amplitude

As we noted above, the value 0 in the graph in Figure 3.2 corresponds to the height that the water would have if there were no waves. The vertical scale has negative values that correspond to water levels below this height, and positive values for water levels above this height. Note that the high and low points for each cycle of the waveform in Figure 3.2 have the same numerical value, 2 feet. The waveform plotted in Figure 3.2 is a sinusoidal waveform. The *amplitude* of a wave is, by definition, the maximum or minimum deviation from the zero line. The amplitude of the sine wave in Figure 3.2 is 2 feet. The amplitude of a wave essentially is a measure of its size. The amplitude is independent of the frequency of the wave. The greater the amplitude, the "bigger" the wave. One can have either a big or a small ocean wave coming towards the beach during the same time interval (i.e. with the same frequency). Figure 3.3 shows a sinusoidal waveform that has the same frequency as that plotted in 3.2, but half the amplitude.

The waveforms plotted in Figures 3.2 and 3.3 are, as we have noted, *sinusoidal*. Sinusoidal waves, which always have this smooth shape, are important mathematical constructs because it is possible to analyze any complex periodic waveform in terms of a set of sinusoidal waveforms. This is extremely useful since the behavior of devices like organ pipes or the human

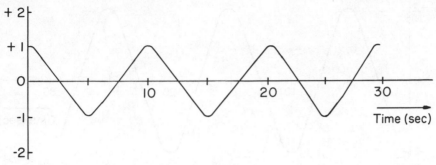

Figure 3.3. Sinusoidal wave, with the same frequency but half the amplitude of that in Figure 3.2.

vocal tract can be calculated in terms of sinusoidal sound sources. Since we may analyze any complex periodic wave in terms of sinusoids, we can thereby predict the response of a device like the human vocal tract to any periodic waveform. We will discuss these procedures later in this chapter. For the moment we will simply note that a sinusoidal waveform can be completely specified by noting its frequency, amplitude, and phase.

Phase

The waveform plotted in Figure 3.2 had a height of + 2 feet when we started to measure it at $t = 0$ second. It had a height of − 2 feet after 5 seconds. Suppose that we had measured a wave that started off at $t = 0$ second with a height of − 2 feet, and this second wave had exactly the same amplitude and period as the wave we actually measured. How could we convey this information? We could, of course, make a graph of the second wave. In Figure 3.4 the graph of this second wave is plotted. Note that this second wave could be obtained by shifting the wave plotted in Figure 3.2 a half period forward. In other words, the wave in Figure 3.3 is equivalent to that of Figure 3.2 shifted by half of its period. The two waves are by definition $\frac{1}{2}$ period *out of phase*.

It is usual to quantify phase differences in terms of degrees. If we divide the total period into 360 degrees, then $\frac{1}{2}$ period equals 180 degrees, and the two waves plotted in Figure 3.2 and 3.4 are 180 degrees out of phase.

The human auditory system is not very sensitive to phase. Slight shifts in the phase of a waveform are not usually perceptible, although large shifts can be heard. Telephone systems traditionally have been designed with this tolerance in mind because it simplifies some of the electronics and saves money. (In recent years the introduction of electronic data transmission devices that, unlike the human auditory system, *are* sensitive to phase differences has made changes in the telephone system's design necessary.)

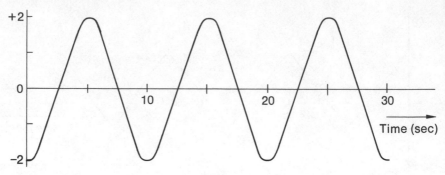

Figure 3.4. Wave of Figure 3.2 shifted in phase.

Wave motion – propagation velocity

When you hit a ball with a baseball bat, you are transferring the energy that you built up by your swing from the bat to the ball. Wave motions are characterized by the transfer of energy. For example, energy is transmitted by an ocean wave when it hits you. The motion of an ocean wave can easily be observed as it sweeps in toward a pier. The crest of the wave moves in with a certain speed. This speed is called the *propagation velocity* of the wave. The propagation velocity of an ocean wave could be determined by observing its crest. In Figure 3.5 we have sketched the crest of an ocean wave at two instants of time at the pier separated by 5 seconds. We could have obtained these data by taking two flash pictures of the scene. The horizontal scale in these pictures is the distance measured in feet from the end of the pier. The vertical scale is the height of the wave. Note that the crest that is at 5 feet in Figure 3.5A is at 0 feet in Figure 3.5B. The velocity of propagation is therefore 1 foot per second (ft/sec).

The fact that the crest has moved does not mean that any molecule of water actually moved 5 feet towards the pier. The energy in the wave has moved forward through the medium of the water. The wave that hits you at the beach at Atlantic City, New Jersey, may, for example, have started from the coast of Portugal, but no molecule of "Portuguese water" will touch you.

It is important to keep in mind the distinction between the transfer of energy in a wave and the motion of the particles of the medium. One traditional demonstration makes use of three coins placed on a table. If the coins are placed in a row and the coin on one end of the row is flipped against the center coin, the energy of the collision will be transmitted to the coin on the other end of the line. The center coin will not move very far. The first coin obviously will not move around the center coin. The energy derived from the motion of the first coin will, however, be transmitted through the middle coin to the last coin. The point to keep in mind is that the energy that was originally in the first coin

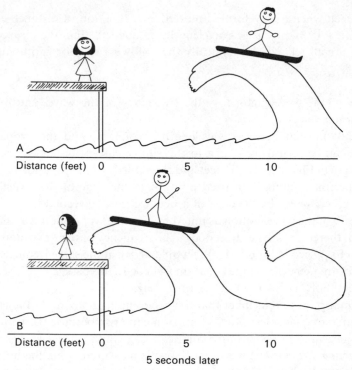

A

Distance (feet) 0   5   10

B

Distance (feet) 0   5   10

5 seconds later

Figure 3.5. Propagation of an ocean wave. (A) At first measurement. (B) 5 seconds later.

transferred to the third coin, although the first coin never actually touched the third coin.

The transmission of energy in a sound wave is like the transmission of energy through the row of coins. The molecules of gas that form the atmosphere transmit forces as they collide with each other. The sound that you hear has been transmitted by a wave that has exerted a pressure on your eardrums. In a near vacuum, as in outer space or the moon, where there are no gas molecules, sound cannot be transmitted. The pressure that a sound wave exerts is no different from the pressure that is exerted on your finger when you press it down against the open end of an open water faucet. The water actually pushes against your finger. It exerts a certain force per unit area. A sound wave exerts a force against your eardrums.

In Figure 3.5B the crest of a second cycle of the wave has been drawn. Note that the distance between the two crests of the periodic wave motion is 10 feet. The wavelength of the periodic wave is thus 10 feet. The *wavelength* is, by definition, the distance between recurring events in a wave motion distributed over distance. The wavelength is *not* the same as the period. The wavelength

23

can be seen when a waveform is plotted as a function of distance *at some particular instant of time*. Wavelength, frequency, and the propagation velocity are all related. Algebraically the following relationship holds:

$$\lambda f = c$$

where λ = the wavelength, f = the frequency of the wave, and c = the propagation velocity.

The relationship between wavelength, frequency, and the propagation velocity can be seen if we return to the simple case of ocean waves. If the wavelength in Figure 3.5B is 10 feet and the velocity of propagation is 1 ft/sec, then a person standing at a fixed point, e.g., the edge of the beach at the waterline, will be hit by the crest of a new wave at 10-second intervals. The periodicity of the wave motion as noted by the observer standing at this fixed location, therefore, will be 10 seconds. The frequency of the wave motion will be equal to $\frac{1}{10}$ second, or 0.1 Hz. We would arrive at the same frequency if we solved for frequency using the equation $f = c/\lambda$. In this case, c = 1 ft/sec and λ = 10 feet. Solving for f, we get $\frac{1}{10}$ or 0.1 Hz.

It is important to remember that the wavelength and period of a wave are quite different quantities. Much confusion can arise because the period of a wave is measured along the horizontal scale of a graph when a wave is plotted *as a function of time*. The wavelength also is measured along the horizontal scale of a graph when a wave is plotted *as a function of distance*. In one case the horizontal axis is measuring the course of time at a fixed location. In the other case the horizontal scale is measuring the amplitude of the wave along the dimension of distance for a particular instant of time.

Fourier analysis

At first glance there would appear to be very little in common between sinusoidal waveforms like that plotted in Figure 3.2 and the waveform plotted in Figure 3.5. A fundamental principle of mathematics, however, shows that it is always possible to analyze a "complex" periodic waveform like that of Figure 3.5 into a set of sinusoidal waveforms. Any periodic waveform, no matter how complex it is, can be closely approximated by adding together a number of sinusoidal waveforms. The mathematical procedure of *Fourier analysis* tells us what particular set of sinusoids go together to make up a particular complex waveform. We won't go into the details of Fourier analysis except to note the important fact that the set of sinusoids that one adds together to approximate a particular complex waveform are harmonically related. What does this mean?

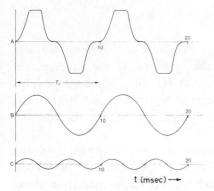

Figure 3.6. (A) A complex waveform. (B) and (C) Its first two sinusoidal Fourier components.

Fundamental frequency (f_0)

In Figure 3.6A we have plotted a complex waveform and in Figure 3.6B and 3.6C its first two sinusoidal Fourier components. All three graphs have the same horizontal time scale and same vertical amplitude scale. The complex waveform could, for example, be the sound waveform recorded by a microphone monitoring a loudspeaker. Note that the complex waveform, A, is *not* sinusoidal. Its leading edge, for example, rises sharply; it has a flat top, etc. It is, however, a periodic waveform and the duration of its period is, as Figure 3.6 shows, 10 milliseconds. As noted in an earlier chapter, milliseconds are convenient units for the measurement of the periods of audible sound waves. The first two sinusoidal components, B and C, are plotted beneath the complex waveform. The period of waveform B, the first component, is equal to the period T_0 of the complex waveform. This is always the case. This period, which is the time in seconds that it takes for the complex waveform to repeat itself, is called the *fundamental period*. The frequency of the first component is called the *fundamental frequency*. The frequency of the first component always is equal to the frequency of the complex wave. The symbol f_0 is usually used to represent the fundamental frequency. Algebraically:

$$f_0 = \frac{1}{T_0} = \frac{1}{T}$$

Thus, solving the equation, the fundamental frequency of the complex wave in Figure 3.6 is

$$\frac{1}{0.01 \text{ sec}} = 100 \text{ Hz}$$

25

Harmonics

One of the discoveries of Fourier analysis was that the components of a complex wave are related in a predictable manner. If the fundamental frequency f_0 of a wave is, for example, 100 Hz, then the next possible component, the *first harmonic*, has a frequency of two times f_0, i.e. 200 Hz. The second harmonic has a frequency of three times f_0, i.e. 300 Hz, the next one four times, and so on.

In the periodic waveform and components sketched in Figure 3.6B, the frequency of the first harmonic is 100 Hz. The frequency of the second harmonic, Figure 3.6C, is 200 Hz. To achieve a better approximation of the complex waveform it would be necessary to add other components that had still higher frequencies to the sum of the first two sinusoids. The frequencies of these higher sinusoidal components would all be harmonically related to the fundamental frequency. The frequency of the third sinusoidal component, for example, would be equal to $3f_0$; the frequency of the fourth component would be $4f_0$; etc. The frequency of the nth component would be equal to nf_0.

Adult human beings can generally perceive sounds from 20 to about 15 000 Hz. That means that human listeners can hear the sinusoidal components of complex sounds for frequencies between 20 and 15 000 Hz. Children and many young adults can hear frequencies higher than 15 000 Hz. The upper limit is generally about 20 000 Hz, but it falls with age. The meaningful sinusoidal components that constitute human speech are, for the most part, below 7000 Hz; hence, telephone systems that transmit frequencies no higher than 5000 Hz are adequate for most purposes (Flanagan, 1972).

Spectrum

In the Fourier analysis of a complex waveform the amplitude of each sinusoidal component depends on the shape of the particular complex wave. It is therefore necessary to keep track of the amplitude of each component if one wants to specify a complex wave in terms of its sinusoidal components. The mathematical procedures for determining the amplitudes of the Fourier components of a complex wave involve difficult calculations and will not be described here. Computer programs have been designed for the analysis of complex waves that can quickly make these calculations. We can conveniently keep track of the frequencies and amplitudes of the sinusoidal components that go together to make up a complex wave by means of graphs like that in Figure 3.7.

The horizontal axis is the frequency scale (note 1 kHz (kilohertz) = 1000 Hz); the vertical axis is the amplitude scale. The amplitude of each component

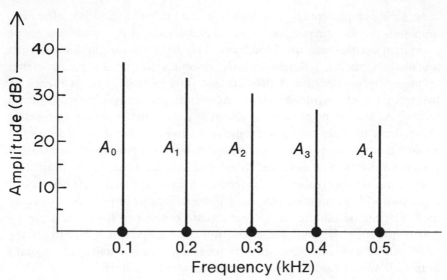

Figure 3.7. Graph of a spectrum.

is represented by a line at the frequency of each sinusoidal component. This type of graph is known as a graph of the spectrum. We have plotted the amplitudes of the first two sinusoidal components shown in Figure 3.6 as well as the next three higher components. Note that the graph consists of vertical lines at each sinusoidal frequency. This signifies that there is sound energy present *only* at these discrete frequencies. We did not connect the data points because there physically is *no* energy present at any frequency between the harmonics. This type of spectrum is sometimes called a *line* spectrum. It differs from spectra that have energy distributed over a broad, continuous range of frequencies.

We have not kept track of the parameter called *phase* that we would need if we were actually to add up a number of sinusoidal components to make up a particular complex waveform. Phase, as we noted, is not particularly important in the perception of speech. The conceptual value of representing a complex waveform as a spectrum will be apparent in Chapter 4.

Amplitude and frequency scales for speech

The perceptually relevent metric for the amplitude of a speech wave is its pressure. When we say that one sound is "louder" than another we usually are responding to the relative amplitudes of the two sounds. Loudness is our *perceptual* response to the amplitude of the speech signal. When we listen to short sounds lasting under 500 milliseconds, the duration of the sound also

27

influences our perceptual judgement of loudness (c.f. p. 154). However, amplitude, i.e. the air pressure of the speech signal, is the primary acoustic "correlate" of the percept of loudness. This follows from the fact that the mammalian auditory system directly responds to the air pressure that impinges on the eardrum. A pressure is a force per unit area. A higher air pressure pushes the eardrum in more, a lower air pressure pushes the eardrum in less. As the air pressure of a sound wave fluctuates above and below atmospheric pressure, the eardrum moves in and out. By means of a series of anatomical and electrophysiological mechanisms, the motion of the eardrum is transformed into an electrical signal that is transmitted to the brain.

Pressures are always measured in terms of a force per unit area. If you look at a gas station's tire pressure gauge it will be calibrated in pounds per square inch. The metric units of dynes per square centimetre (dyne/cm^2) are by convention the basic units for speech signals. However, it is rare to see the amplitude of a speech signal directly measured in these units. The signal's amplitude will instead be given in decibels, abbreviated dB.

The decibel is a logarithmic unit. Logarithmic units relate quantities in terms of the "power" ratios. The logarithmic ratio between a sound pressure of 1000 dyne/cm^2 and one of 10 dyne/cm^2 would be equal to 2 if we took the log to the base 10, i.e. $\frac{1000}{10}$ which equals 10^2. The logarithm is the power 2, the number of times that the base, 10, would have to be multiplied by itself. It is obvious that a logarithmic scale would be useful if we had to make a graph of a function that encompassed a great range. If a sound pressure varied over a range of 10 to 1000 dyne/cm^2, it would be difficult to plot the range on any reasonable sized paper. If we, for example, plotted this range of amplitude variation using a scale value of 1 mm for each dyne/cm^2, the graph would be a metre high. If we wanted to be able to plot a range of amplitudes that corresponded to the total dynamic range of the human auditory system we would need a graph that was about 100 metres high. If we convert sound pressures to a logarithmic scale, it becomes feasible to plot the range of amplitude values that are relevant for human speech.

The decibel is defined in terms of a fixed air pressure reference. It is equal to

$$20 \log_{10} \frac{P}{0.0002 \text{ dyne/cm}^2}$$

where P = the pressure measured. All sounds are measured in relation to this basic reference point. It is not necessary to memorize this number because relative values are what are usually important. The decibel scale is a convenient scale for the measurement of sound since it is a relative scale. Some useful indices to what various decibel measurements "mean" perceptually can follow from the following examples of average sound pressures:

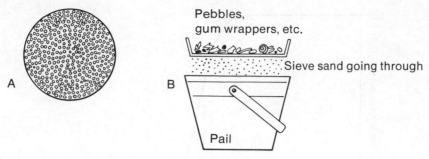

Figure 3.8. Sieve as mechanical filter. (A) Top view of sieve of average hole diameter d_h. *(B) Side view of sieve in action.*

A "quiet" average room – 30 dB
A noisy average room – 70 dB
A few inches in front of someone shouting – 80 dB
"Inside" a rock band – 100 dB
Ten feet to the side of the rear of a jet engine at full power – 115 dB

A sound perceived as being roughly twice as loud as another is usually about 6 dB greater. The decibel scale is a more suitable scale in terms of perceived loudness than a linear scale. The relative "loudness" of sounds is roughly in accord with a logarithmic or "power" scale to the human auditory system (Flanagan, 1972). There are differences between a logarithmic and power scale, but these differences are not particularly germane to our understanding of the perception of speech.

Filters

In the next chapter we will discuss speech production in terms of the source–filter theory. Before we discuss this theory, which involves an understanding of some of the specific properties of acoustic filters, we will briefly introduce some of the general properties of filters. Perhaps the simplest example of a filter is a sieve or strainer, so we will return to our hypothetical demonstration site at the beach where we looked at ocean waves. This time we will stay on the sand for our examples and examine some of the general properties of filters as they are exemplified in the properties of beach sieves.

Figure 3.8A shows what we would see if we looked down at the top of a child's sieve. We would see a pattern of holes, each with approximately the same diameter. Let us call this diameter d_h, the average hole diameter. Obviously the holes will not all have exactly the same diameter – children's beach sieves are not precision-made.

Sand particles of diameters less than that of the holes in the sieve flow through the sieve into the child's pail below. Larger objects like pebbles, candy

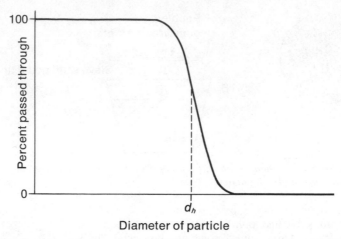

Figure 3.9. Transfer function of sieve as "small-diameter pass through" filter.

wrappers, and sand particles of large diameter are left in the sieve. The sieve is acting as a mechanical *filter* that affects the transfer of particles into the pail. If the sieve had not been used, all of the large-diameter particles, pebbles, and candy wrappers would have entered the pail. We can quantitatively describe the filtering properties of the sieve placed above the pail by means of the graph in Figure 3.9.

The graph plots the *transfer function* of the sieve. The vertical scale denotes the percent of material that will pass through, i.e. transfer through, the filter. The horizontal scale denotes the size of the particle. The graph thus shows that 100 percent, i.e. all, particles that are very much smaller than the average hole diameter d_h will pass through the sieve. Zero percent of the very large objects will pass through. Particles that have diameters close to the average hole diameter d_h may or may not pass through. It will depend on whether a particular particle is above one of the smaller or one of the bigger holes. Some particles that are larger than the average hole diameter will get through if they happen to be positioned above a hole whose diameter is also larger than the average diameter d_h. Some particles that have smaller diameters will not get through if they are positioned above smaller holes. The filter thus does not abruptly "cut off" the flow of sand at some exact particle diameter; its transfer function instead exhibits a gradual cut-off.

The mechanical filtering system exemplified by the sieve and pail constitute what we would term a "small-diameter pass through" filter. Small particles will go through; bigger particles will be trapped above. We could, using the same pail and sieve, collect the material that was trapped in the filter. If we periodically collected the material trapped in the *top of the sieve* and put that material in the pail, discarding the small particles that flowed through the

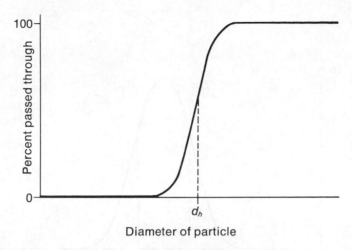

Figure 3.10. Transfer function of sieve as "large-diameter pass through" filter.

sieve, we would have a "large-diameter pass through" filter with the transfer function sketched in Figure 3.10. The same sieve and pail permit us to filter for either large- or small-diameter particles depending on how we arrange them.

We could filter out a small range of particle sizes by sequentially using two different sieves. These different sieves would have to have different average hole diameters. If we first placed the sieve with the larger average hole diameter above the pail, collected the material that accumulated in the pail, and then poured this material through the sieve with the smaller diameter, we would be left with particles *in the sieve* that were restricted to a small range or "band" of diameters. The transfer function plotted in Figure 3.11 quantitatively represents the result of this sequential process for a case where the average hole diameters of the two sieves are close, although not identical, in size. Note that maximum transfer through the complete filter system occurs about particle diameter d_c and that there exists a range of particle sizes d_w for which most e.g. 70 percent, will get through the filter system to be collected.

We have presented this discussion of the filtering properties of beach sieves and pails because the supralaryngeal vocal tract – the air passages of the mouth, pharynx, and nose – acts as an adjustable acoustic filter that allows certain bands of wavelengths of sound to pass through. Wavelength-sensitive filters are analogous to the particle diameter "band pass" filter whose transfer function is sketched in Figure 3.11.

The discussion of mechanical filters can be applied to the filtering action of the vocal tract. The supralaryngeal vocal tract is a wavelength-sensitive acoustic filter. We can therefore describe its properties by noting the wavelengths at which maximum sound energy will pass through, as well as the

31

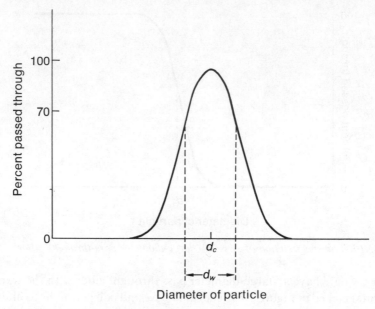

Figure 3.11. Transfer function of two sieves used to make a "band pass" filter.

range of wavelengths that will mostly get through (the acoustic analogs of d_c and d_w.) The product of the wavelength and frequency of a wave is equal to the propagation velocity (the algebraic relationship $\lambda f = c$). The velocity of sound, c, is constant in air under normal conditions. It is therefore appropriate to describe the transfer function of the supralaryngeal vocal tract filter in terms of frequency. The *center frequencies* at which maximum sound energy will pass through the filter systems are called *formant frequencies*. We will discuss the supralaryngeal vocal tract filter in the following chapters because the controlled variation of formant frequencies is perhaps the single most important factor in human speech.

Exercises

1.   Suppose that the temperature pattern plotted in Figure 3.1 prevailed over a few weeks yielding a quasi-periodic weather pattern.

(a) What is the fundamental frequency of the waveform plotted in Figure 3.1?
(b) What is the frequency of the first harmonic of this waveform?
(c) Would the Fourier components that make up the waveform plotted in Figure 3.1 be sinusoids?

2.   Plot the Fourier spectrum of the complex waveform plotted in Figure 3.6A. Make a graph similar to that of Figure 3.7. What is the amplitude and

frequency of the first component? What is the amplitude of the second component?

3. Copy the transfer function plotted in Figure 3.11. Draw over this plot, using dashed red lines, the transfer function as a "new" band pass filter. The "new" filter has the same d_c as the "old" filter plotted in Figure 3.11. However, the new filter's d_w, its "bandwidth," is twice that of the old filter.

4. Given that the velocity of sound in air is approximately 1100 feet per second, what would be the frequency of a sound with a wavelength of 20 feet?

5. If the period of a complex waveform is 20 milliseconds, what is its fundamental frequency?

4

Source–filter theory of speech production

In this chapter we will discuss the basic aspects of the source-filter theory of speech production that we introduced in Chapter 2. In the chapters that follow we will consider the acoustic characteristics that differentiate many of the sounds of speech and the articulatory gestures that underlie speech. The source–filter theory makes it possible to relate the acoustic and articulatory levels in a quantitative and coherent manner.

The laryngeal source

Let us start by considering the production of a *voiced* sound, i.e. one in which the vocal cords interrupt the air flow from the lungs, producing *phonation*. The larynx can serve as a source of sound energy. It can produce a periodic wave through the process of phonation, as for example in the word *mama*. It can also generate a "noise" source, e.g. the source during the [h] sound of *Hop!* The source of sound energy when we whisper is the noise generated through air turbulence at the glottal constriction. The vocal cords do not have to move during a whisper. Many of the sounds of speech involve sources of sound that are generated through turbulent air flow through constrictions at other parts of the airways of the vocal tract. However, it will be useful to begin our discussion of the source–filter theory of speech production by considering voiced sounds in which the larynx produces a periodic source.

During phonation, the vocal cords rapidly open and close in a quasi-periodic fashion. As they open and close, air flows through the opening. More air will flow through when the opening is greater, and less air when the opening is smaller. Figure 4.1 shows three cycles of this air flow pattern. Note that the period of the complex waveform is 0.01 second or 10 milliseconds. The fundamental frequency of this periodic glottal air flow is thus

$$\frac{1}{T} = \frac{1}{0.01 \ \text{sec}} = 100 \ \text{Hz}$$

The spectrum of this glottal air flow is plotted in Figure 4.2. Note that the glottal spectrum shows that the waveform of Figure 4.1 has energy at the

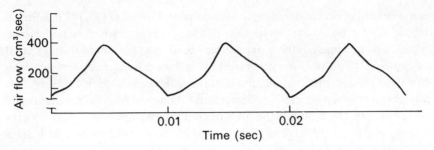

Figure 4.1. *Three cycles of a waveform typical of the air flow through the glottis during phonation.*

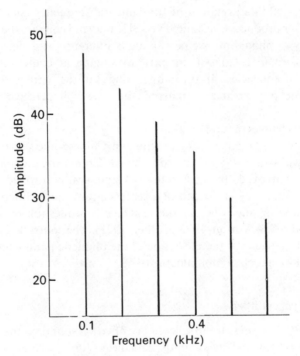

Figure 4.2. *Spectrum of typical glottal air flow.*

fundamental frequency (100 Hz = 0.1 kHz) and at higher harmonics. Note also that the amplitude of the harmonics gradually falls. This is a general property of the laryngeal source. We have not drawn the complete spectrum, but there is perceptible acoustic energy up to at least 3000 Hz present in the typical glottal air flow of a male speaker phonating at a fundamental frequency of 100 Hz.

The rate at which the vocal cords open and close during phonation determines the period and, hence, the fundamental frequency (f_0) of the glottal air flow. Within broad limits a speaker can vary this rate, which is determined by the shape and mass of the moving vocal cords, the tension of the laryngeal muscles, and the air pressure generated by the lungs. Adult male speakers can phonate at fundamental frequencies that range between 80 and 300 Hz. Adult females and children normally phonate at fundamental frequencies that range up to about 500 Hz, although the fundamental frequency can go up to 1.5 kHz (Keating and Buhr, 1978). The longer vocal cords of adult males, which are a consequence of secondary sexual dimorphism in *Homo sapiens*, yield a lower range of fundamental frequencies. (The thyroid cartilage grows differentially during puberty in males, cf. Kirchner, 1970, pp. 15–17.)

The perceptual interpretation of fundamental frequency is *pitch*. When a human speaker produces a sustained vowel sound and changes the fundamental frequency of phonation, we perceive the difference as a change in pitch. Musical performances consist, in part, of singing at controlled, specified fundamental frequencies. If the singer sings at the wrong fundamental frequency, the performance is marred since we will perceive it as being "offpitch."

Controlled changes in fundamental frequency also can be used for linguistic purposes. In many languages, for example in Chinese, the same vowels and consonants will signify different words when different fundamental frequency patterns are employed. In most human languages, controlled changes in fundamental frequency at the end of a sentence can signify differences in the sentence's meaning, e.g. whether the sentence is a question or a statement (Lieberman, 1967; Atkinson, 1973; Collier, 1975). The controlled variation of fundamental frequency is therefore one of the phonetic parameters that may be employed in speech communication.

The supralaryngeal filter

A trained singer can sing an entire sequence of vowel sounds at the same pitch. The differences between vowel sounds, called *vowel quality*, are independent of the activity of the larynx. They are the consequences of changes in the shape of the supralaryngeal airway. During the production of human speech the shape of the supralaryngeal airway continually changes. The supralaryngeal airway always acts as an acoustic filter, suppressing the transfer of sound energy at certain frequencies, letting maximum energy through at other frequencies. The frequencies at which local energy maxima may pass through the supralaryngeal air passages are called *formant frequencies*. The formant frequencies are determined by the length and shape of the supralaryngeal vocal tract, which acts as an acoustic filter. The larynx and subglottal system have

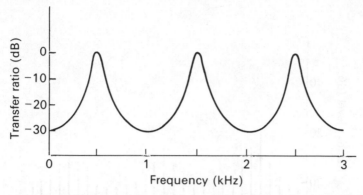

Figure 4.3. Transfer function of the supralaryngeal vocal tract for the vowel [ə]. For our purposes, the term "transfer function" is equivalent to "filter function." Note the locations of the formant frequencies at 0.5, 1.5, and 2.5 kHz.

only minor effects on the formant frequencies (Fant, 1960; Flanagan, 1972). Vowels like [a], [i], [æ], and [ʌ] owe their phonetic quality to their different formant frequencies.

In Figure 4.3 we have plotted the "transfer function" of the supralaryngeal airway for the vowel [ə] (the first vowel in the word *about*). This is the idealized supralaryngeal filter function for a speaker having a supralaryngeal vocal tract of approximately 17 cm. The length of the supralaryngeal vocal tract for this vowel would be measured along the centerline of the air passage from the lips to the glottal opening of the larynx, excluding the nasal cavity (Fant, 1960). The formant frequencies for this vowel are 500, 1500, and 2500 Hz. The symbols F_1, F_2, F_3 are usually used to denote the formant frequencies of speech sounds. F_1 denotes the lowest formant frequency, which is 500 Hz in this example; F_2, the second formant, 1500 Hz in this example, etc. The formant frequencies are essentially the center frequencies of the supralaryngeal vocal tract acting as a complex filter that lets maximum sound energy through in several bands of frequency. The frequency bands of each formant have an appreciable bandwidth, from 60 to 100 Hz. Other vowels would have different formant frequencies and bandwidths. The formant frequencies of the vowel [i], for example, would be about 240 Hz for F_1, 2200 Hz for F_2, and 5200 Hz for F_3 for this particular speaker. The first three formants of vowels play the major role in specifying these sounds. Higher formants exist, but they are not necessary for the perception of vowel differences. The bandwidths of the formants of different vowels also do not markedly distinguish different vowels (Fant, 1960; Flanagan, 1972).

In Figure 4.4 we have plotted the spectrum that would result if the laryngeal source with the spectrum plotted in Figure 4.2 were filtered by the transfer

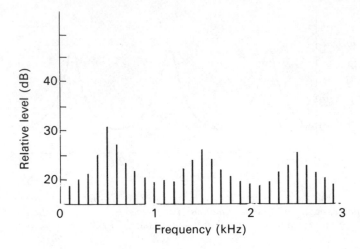

Figure 4.4. The spectrum that would result if the transfer function plotted in Figure 4.3 were "excited" by the glottal source plotted in Figure 4.2. The sound is the vowel [ə].

function plotted in Figure 4.3. The resulting spectrum would describe the speech signal measured at the end of the air passages of the vocal tract. Note that sound energy would be present at each of the harmonics of the glottal source, but the amplitude of each harmonic would be a function of *both* the filter function and the amplitude of the particular harmonic of the glottal source. A human listener hearing a speech signal having the spectrum plotted in Figure 4.4 would recognize the signal as a token of the vowel [ə] that had a fundamental frequency of 100 Hz. In Figure 4.5 we have plotted a stylized speech waveform that would correspond to the spectrum of Figure 4.4. Unlike Figure 4.4, Figure 4.5 is a plot of the air pressure as a function of time. More realistic waveforms that show the period-to-period variations of the glottal source will be discussed in Chapter 5. Note that the waveform plotted in Figure 4.5 resembles the glottal source waveform that was plotted in Figure 4.1 only in so far as it has the same period and frequency (0.01 sec and 100 Hz). The interposition of the supralaryngeal vocal tract has modified the glottal waveform and we can see that the laryngeal source is only one factor in the production of speech. The source–filter theory of speech, which formally takes account of these two factors, the source and the filter, was first proposed by Johannes Müller (1848). It has been developed on a quantitative basis in recent years. Studies like those of Chiba and Kajiyama (1941), Fant (1960), and Stevens and House (1955) make possible a quantitative prediction of the filtering effects of particular configurations of the supralaryngeal air passages.

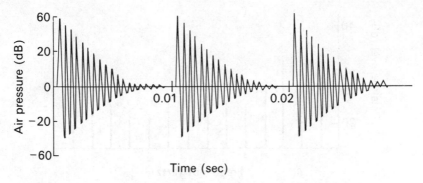

Figure 4.5. Speech waveform as measured by a microphone sensitive to air pressure variations. The human ear is itself sensitive to air pressure variations.

The perception of fundamental and formant frequencies

The perception of speech in human beings appears to involve specialized neural mechanisms. The perception of fundamental frequency by the human brain appears to be made primarily through waveform measurements that derive the period (Flanagan, 1972). The neural procedures used in making these measurements appear to be fairly complex and they can be simulated only through the use of elaborate computer programs (Gold, 1962). The computer program has to "know" (i.e. the programmer must insert subroutines that take account of) the variation in the rate of change of fundamental frequency that normally occurs from one period to the next (Lieberman, 1961). The computer program must also "know" how different supralaryngeal vocal tract transfer functions will affect the speech waveform; it must "know" the probable variations in the glottal spectrum that can occur at the onset and end of phonation as the larynx responds to transient conditions in air flow, air pressure, and laryngeal muscle tension. Despite the persistent application of the most advanced engineering techniques, a satisfactory "pitch extractor" is still not available, although there have been important commercial applications since 1937 (Flanagan, 1972).

The procedures that the brains of human listeners use in deriving the formant frequencies of speech from the acoustic signal appear to be even more complex. These perceptual "recognition procedures" must involve the analysis of the speech signal in terms of its spectrum, but they go far beyond the simple examination of a spectrum for local energy maxima. The formant frequencies plotted in Figure 4.3 show up in Figure 4.4 as local peaks at 500, 1500, and 2500 Hz because the fundamental frequency f_0 is 100 Hz. Thus, there are harmonics at each of the formant frequencies. However, this is not always the case. If you excited the same supralaryngeal vocal tract configuration, e.g.

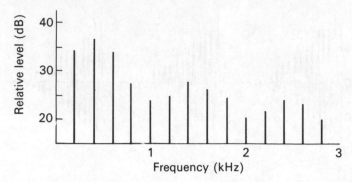

Figure 4.6. Spectrum of the sound [ə] produced with a different fundamental frequency of phonation. The speech signal still has the phonetic quality of the vowel [ə] although it has a different fundamental frequency than the [ə] whose spectrum is plotted in Figure 4.4.

for the schwa vowel [ə] with a different fundamental frequency, the spectrum of the sound [ə] would be different. Figure 4.6 shows the spectrum for the vowel [ə] with a fundamental frequency of 200 Hz. Note that the peaks in the spectrum occur at 400, 1400, and 2400 Hz. However, the formant frequencies of Figures 4.4 and 4.6 are actually the same, and a human listener would perceive both sounds as being the vowel [ə].

The listener would have to deduce the location of the formant frequencies from a spectrum that actually lacked peaks at the formants. Formant frequencies are not always directly manifested in the acoustic signal that has been filtered by the supralaryngeal vocal tract. The formant frequencies are really the frequencies at which the supralaryngeal filter *would* let maximum energy through (Hermann, 1894). If the glottal source lacks acoustic energy at a particular formant frequency then there will be *no* acoustic energy in the output signal at that frequency. The graphs plotted in Figure 4.7 illustrate this point. Graph A is a line spectrum of a glottal source with a fundamental frequency of 500 Hz. This is a possible fundamental frequency for many children and some adult women. Graph B is a transfer function of the vowel [i]. The formant frequencies are appropriate for an adult female (Peterson and Barney, 1952). Graph C is a plot of the speech signal that results from the filtering of the 500 Hz fundamental frequency source by the [i] filter. Note that there is no energy at the formant frequencies marked by the circled X's in graph C.

The electronic instrument that in the past was most often used for the analysis of speech, the sound spectrograph, will not "show" formant frequencies for signals like the one represented in graph C of Figure 4.7 (Koenig, Dunn and Lacey, 1946). The most recent computer-implemented

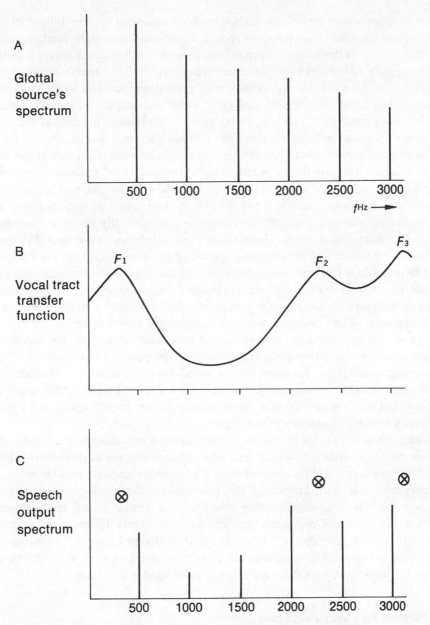

Figure 4.7. (A) Spectrum of glottal source. (B) Transfer function for vowel [i]. (C) Spectrum of the speech signal that would result if transfer function (B) were excited by glottal source (A). Note that the formant frequencies of the transfer function are not directly manifested in the speech signal by acoustic energy at the points labeled X.

41

techniques, which we will discuss in Chapter 5, also tend to have difficulties in deriving formant frequencies for speech signals that have high fundamental frequencies. In contrast, the perception of speech in human listeners is only marginally affected by high fundamental frequencies. Error rates increase very slightly as the fundamental frequency of phonation increases when listeners are asked to identify vowels that differ only with respect to their formant frequency patterns (Ryalls and Lieberman, 1982). Human listeners appear to derive formant frequencies through a procedure that makes use of their unconscious, internalized knowledge of the mechanisms and physics of speech production. It is possible to program digital computers to "recognize" vowels using this sort of procedure (Bell *et al.*, 1961). The computer program has access to a memory in which the acoustic consequences of various possible vocal tract shapes are stored. The computer systematically generates internal spectra using this memory. The internally generated spectra are then matched against the spectra of the incoming speech signal. The process does not select the individual formant frequencies on the basis of a single local energy maximum, but rather on the match between the total spectrum of the incoming speech signal and the internally generated signal specified by all three formant frequencies. The computer program is relatively complex because it must model the performance of human listeners who appear to have neural mechanisms that are especially adapted to the perception of speech. The computer program, for example, "knows" that the relative amplitude of formant peaks for vowels is determined by the value of each formant frequency and that the overall shape of the spectrum is thus largely specified by the positions of the formants (Fant, 1956).

Speech scientists are able to use computers and instruments like the sound spectrograph to derive formant frequencies by making use of their knowledge of where the formant frequencies of various sounds *should* be. In other words, they make use of the knowledge that has been acquired by looking at a great many speech samples when they interpret a particular sound spectrogram (Cole *et al.*, 1980). Despite this prior knowledge, it is very difficult to determine the formant frequencies of a signal like that plotted in Figure 4.7, although a human listener will have no difficulty in recognizing the vowel. We will return to this topic when we discuss the analysis of speech in Chapter 5.

Formant frequency calculation

We have stated that the shape and length of the supralaryngeal air passages cause them to act as an acoustic filter. Although the calculations that are necessary to determine the transfer function that corresponds to a particular supralaryngeal vocal tract shape often are complex and difficult to follow, the

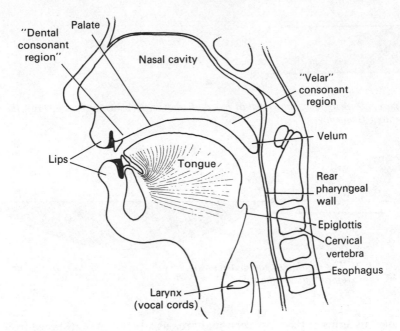

Figure 4.8. The adult human vocal tract.

relationship between the vocal tract shape and the formant frequencies is straightforward and simple in some cases. It is useful to get an appreciation or "feel" for the problem from these simple cases since the general principles that govern the relationship between vocal tract shape and formant frequencies apply for both simple and complex vocal tract shapes. The physical basis of the relationship between the formant frequencies and the shape and size of the supralaryngeal vocal tract is perhaps easiest to see for the unnasalized vowel [ə].

The vowel [ə] called schwa (the first vowel in the word *about*) is perhaps the "simplest" and most basic vowel sound. The sketch in Figure 4.8 shows a stylized midsagittal view of the supralaryngeal vocal tract as derived from X-ray movies of speech for this vowel. The speaker's velum is raised, closing the nasal cavity off from the rest of the supralaryngeal airways. The speaker's lips are neither advanced nor retracted. The speaker's tongue is in a fairly unperturbed position with respect to the shape that it assumes during quiet respiration (Perkell, 1969).

Any point in the vocal tract has a cross-sectional area. The manner in which the cross-sectional area varies along the length of the vocal tract (the area function) determines the formant frequencies. In this case, the area function is acoustically equivalent to a uniform tube open at one end. The area function is

43

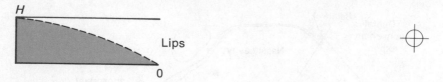

Figure 4.9. A uniform tube open at one end, showing a pressure waveform at the first formant frequency.

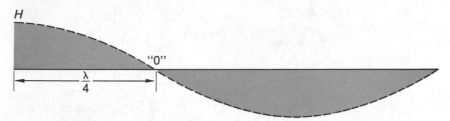

Figure 4.10. The relation of the quarter-wavelength "inside" the tube to the air pressure waveform outside the tube.

plotted in terms of the cross-sectional area as a function of distance from the glottis. The vocal tract is thus open at the speaker's lips. The glottis is represented as a complete closure because the average glottal opening is quite small during normal phonation. The speaker's nasal cavity would be sealed by the velum during the production of an unnasalized vowel so we have only one tube in the supralaryngeal airway for the vowel [ə]. The supralaryngeal vocal tract for this vowel behaves rather like an organ pipe and we can see how the formant frequencies are related to the shape and length, i.e. the area function of the pipe.

In Figure 4.9 we have sketched a uniform pipe open at one end. We have superimposed on the sketch of the pipe a dotted line that represents the pressure waveform of the lowest frequency sinusoidal sound wave that could be sustained in this tube. Sound waves are air pressure waves. At a given instant of time a sinusoidal air pressure wave will be distributed in space. It will have a peak pressure at one point, zero pressure at a distance of one-quarter wavelength from the maximum, a peak pressure at one wavelength from the first peak, etc. We have sketched a pressure wave, marking these points in Figure 4.10. How does the pressure waveform sketched in Figure 4.9 relate to the waveform sketched in Figure 4.10?

Let us imagine that we are trying to "match" the physical constraints of the pipe sketched in Figure 4.9 with the power required to sustain a sinusoidal air pressure wave. In other words, we are trying to take advantage of the physical characteristics of the pipe to minimize the amount of power (or energy) that we would need to generate an air pressure wave. The pressure in an air pressure wave comes from the constant collision of the air molecules. It is obvious that maximum air pressure could most easily be sustained at the closed end of the tube where air molecules would bounce off the rigid wall of the tube to hit other molecules. The letter *H* therefore represents the position of the highest air pressure in Figure 4.9. The walls and closed end of the tube, the "boundaries," aid in maintaining a high air pressure because they constrain the air molecules and build up the number of collisions between the air molecules as they bounce off the closed end.

A useful physical analogy is to imagine the collisions of the air molecules as though these molecules were tennis balls. If the tennis balls were bouncing off a solid wall at the end of the tube they obviously would be more likely to hit each other than if there were no wall. The pressure generated in a gas follows from the collisions between the molecules, thus where there are more collisions the pressure will be higher.

The open end of the tube presents the reverse situation, air molecules simply sail off into the outside world. The air pressure at the end of the tube is "constrained" only by the pressure of the atmosphere outside the tube. Atmospheric pressure is, by definition, zero pressure (negative pressures are pressures below atmospheric). It is obvious that, in the absence of any sound, the air pressure outside of the tube would be at atmospheric pressure. It logically would be easiest to sustain an air pressure wave that had "zero pressure," i.e. just atmospheric pressure, at the open end of the tube. The label 0 therefore appears in Figure 4.9 at the open end of the tube. Note that the examples that we have used to explain the basis for the *H* and 0 pressure points are quite simple. We could use any of a number of other simple examples; 20 people bouncing balls off a wall would be hit more often by the balls than 20 people throwing balls off the end of a ship. The examples can be simple because the physical principle that we are attempting to illustrate is also simple. It is that the boundaries of the tube provide "constraints" that best match certain air pressures. Open ends best match the atmospheric pressure while a closed end will match a pressure maximum.

The question is now whether there exists a sinusoidal wave that could have its high pressure at the closed end of the tube and also have zero pressure at the open end of the tube. The answer to this rhetorical question is that there are a number of sinusoidal waves that would satisfy these "boundary" conditions. The dashed line in Figure 4.9 represents the sinusoidal wave that has the lowest frequency that could meet these boundary conditions. The distance between points *H* and 0, which is one-quarter of the total wavelength, separates the high point of the wave from the "zero" value.

The tube open at one end thus will lend itself to sustaining a sound wave at a frequency whose wavelength is four times the length of the tube. The physical attributes of the tube – the fact that it has a closed end that is 17 cm away from its open end – make it possible to generate, with minimum energy input an air pressure wave whose wavelength is equal to four times 17 cm. If the glottal source were exciting the tube at the closed end, then it would generate an air pressure wave at the frequency corresponding to this wavelength with minimum input energy. For a given input energy, an air pressure wave would be generated at this frequency with maximum amplitude.

The frequency of the pressure wave at which maximum amplitude will be generated is equal to 500 Hz for a 17 cm tube at sea level in a normal atmosphere. This follows from the relationship that we discussed in Chapter 3, $\lambda f = c$. The velocity of sound in air at sea level is approximately 33 500 cm/sec. Since the length of the tube is 17 cm, the wavelength is four times 17 cm, i.e. 68 cm. The frequency of the wave at which a maximum amplitude will be generated is therefore equal to 33 500/68, or about 500 Hz (the actual value is 493 Hz). This frequency is the first formant frequency, f_1. It is the lowest frequency at which maximum sound energy would be generated by a source at the closed, glottal end of the tube.

Air pressure waves at higher frequencies also would satisfy the boundary conditions of the tube, maximum pressure at the glottis, zero pressure at the open lip end. In Figure 4.11 we have sketched a sinusoidal wave that has three times the frequency of the first formant frequency and that also meets these conditions. Its wavelength would be one-third that of the first formant. The second formant frequency for this tube, which is an idealized model of the vowel [ə], would be approximately 1500 Hz for a supralaryngeal vocal tract that was 17 cm long. The third formant for this tube would be 2500 Hz, five times the first formant frequency. The physical dimensions of the 17 cm tube open at one end thus yield the approximate formant frequency values of $F_1 = 500$ Hz, $F_2 = 1500$ Hz, $F_3 = 2500$ Hz (if you compute these values yourself, you will determine that the actual values are $F_1 = 493$ Hz, $F_2 = 1478$ Hz, and $F_3 = 2463$ Hz). The transfer function of this vowel was plotted in Figure 4.3.

The formant frequencies of a uniform tube open at one end will occur at intervals of

$$\frac{(2k+1)c}{4l} \tag{1}$$

where c is the velocity of sound, l is the length of the tube, and k is an integer (i.e. $k = 0, 1, 2, 3, \ldots$). The first formant equals $c/4l$, the second formant $3c/4l$ and the third formant $5c/4l$. Moreover the tube does not have to be exactly uniform in order for the actual formant frequencies to be computed. A tube shaped like a slightly flared trumpet would have slightly higher formant frequencies (Fant,

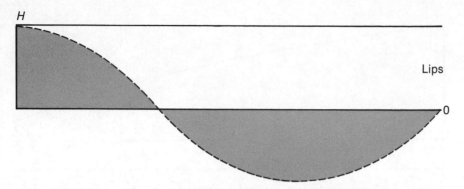

Figure 4.11. The uniform tube of Figure 4.9 showing the second formant frequency, which is three times higher than the first formant frequency.

1960). The walls of the tube could also have slight irregularities and it is not too important what they are made of. Some corrections are necessary in the calculations to take account of the absorption of sound energy by the walls of the tube, but the effects are predictable (Fant, 1960).

Formant frequencies are always determined by the size, length, shape and ends of the supralaryngeal vocal tract, i.e. the cross-sectional area function. As equation (1) above suggests, the formant frequencies will vary as a function of the length of the tube. Now, the average length of a male vocal tract is 17 cm. But what of that of an infant or a woman? Infants' vocal tracts are about one-half the size of men's, whereas women's are about five-sixths. Consequently the formant frequencies of a child or a woman will be considerably higher. For example, the formant frequencies for the vowel [ə] produced by an infant with a vocal tract of 8.5 cm would be approximately 1000 Hz (F_1), 3000 Hz (F_2), and 5000 Hz (F_3).

It is harder to calculate and visualize the physical situation in speech sounds that involve more complex shapes than the vowel [ə]. The formant frequencies are not usually integral multiples of each other and there are some additional factors that influence the total spectrum that we have not considered, e.g. the "radiation impedance" of the lips (Flanagan, 1972). However, the formant frequencies are always determined by the shape and dimensions of the supralaryngeal vocal tract.

Formant lowering and vocal tract length

Suppose that instead of having a fixed-length tube in Figure 4.9 we had a tube whose length was adjustable. If we increased its length while phonation was sustained, the formant frequencies would all fall because the denominator of

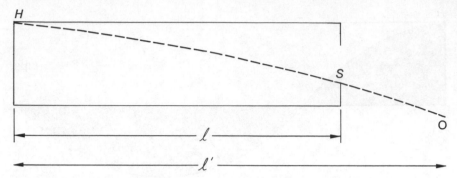

Figure 4.12. Formant frequency lowering that results from a constriction at the end of a uniform tube.

equation (1) would increase. The velocity of sound would be constant so that the formant frequencies would fall as the length of the tube increased. There are two ways in which the human supralaryngeal vocal tract can rapidly increase its length. One of these articulatory gestures is quite obvious. You can protrude your lips. This can add a centimetre or so to the length of the vocal tract (Fant, 1960; Perkell, 1969). The shift in the frequency of F_1 would be about 27 Hz, which would be perceptible to a human listener (Flanagan, 1955a). Traditional phonetic theories are thus correct in claiming that two sounds can be differentiated if the minimal articulatory distinction rests in whether the speakers protrude their lips or not.

Normal human speakers can also lengthen their supralaryngeal vocal tracts by lowering their larynges. In Chapter 6 we will discuss in greater detail the musculature and anatomy of the larynx and the muscles and ligaments that connect it to the rest of the body. The muscles that support and position the larynx can pull it up or down about 2 cm during the production of fluent speech (Perkell, 1969; Ladefoged *et al.*, 1972). If a speaker lowers his larynx 1 cm, the formant frequency shift will be identical to that which would have resulted from a 1 cm protrusion of his lips. The change in length of the supralaryngeal vocal tract is the physiologically relevant phenomenon. If you were listening to this speaker over the telephone or if you were not intently looking at his lips you would not be able to tell how he effected the formant frequency shift. Roman Jakobson stressed the linguistic equivalence of articulatory gestures that have similar acoustic consequences (Jakobson, Fant and Halle, 1963).

The source–filter theory of speech production enables us to evaluate the possible communicative significance of other articulatory gestures. We can, for example, see that the result of constricting the lips by rounding them is acoustically equivalent to lengthening the vocal tract. The sketch of Figure 4.12 shows a uniform tube similar to the previous tubes except for a constriction at its "open" end. The partial block of the open end results in a slight increase in the air pressure behind the constriction. The physical basis for this pressure increase is equivalent to the basis for the increase in pressure that you would feel on your finger as you partially blocked off a water faucet from which water was flowing. The "boundary constraint" for air pressure at the open end thus would best match a pressure S which would be higher than the zero of atmospheric pressure. The dashed line on the sketch is the fraction of a sinusoidal waveform that connects the maximum pressure H with pressure S. Note that this sinusoidal waveform will not reach its zero pressure 0 inside the tube. The wavelength of this sinusoid, which is the lowest frequency sinusoid that can connect the air pressures H and S, is equal to $4(l')$. Since l' is greater than l, the formant frequencies of the tube, which are still determined by equation (1), are lowered. The effect of rounding one's lips[1] is thus equivalent to protruding one's lips, which is again equivalent to lowering one's larynx. The acoustic result of all of these articulatory gestures is *formant frequency lowering*.

The formant frequencies of a uniform tube can likewise be raised by shortening its length. The larynx can move upwards and the lips can be retracted. Both of these gestures can shorten the tube's length, although the lips cannot shorten the vocal tract's length as effectively as they can protrude and lengthen the tube. The lips can open and the jaw can also drop to effectively "flare" the vocal tract and raise the formant frequencies. The extent that the vocal tract can be flared, however, is not as great as the extent to which it can be constricted by closing one's lips. We will return in Chapter 6 to discussing the relationship that holds between the acoustics of speech and particular articulatory maneuvers.

Exercises

1. What would the phonetic quality of the sound produced be for the glottal source shown in Figure 4.7A and supralaryngeal vocal tract configuration of Figure 4.3? Assume that the glottal source is sustained for 200 milliseconds, which corresponds to the duration of a short isolated vowel of English.

2. Consider the glottal source whose spectrum is sketched in Figure 4.7. Is there any acoustic energy present at 700 Hz? Why?

3. Sketch the speech output spectrum for the vocal tract transfer function shown in Figure 4.3 excited by a glottal source of Figure 4.2 which has a fundamental frequency of 100 Hz. Assume that the energy in the harmonics of the fundamental frequency falls off with frequency in a manner similar to the plot in Figure 4.2 i.e. 6 dB per octave. (An octave is a doubling of the frequency; e.g. 100 Hz to 200 Hz is an octave.)

---

[1] The *shape* of the lip constriction is also secondary (Beranek, 1949).

4.   A person who has a supralaryngeal vocal tract 17 cm long maneuvers his tongue, lips, velum, etc. so that the configuration of the vocal tract approximates a uniform tube that changes in length from 17 cm to 20 cm while phonation is sustained. Calculate and sketch the first three formant frequencies as a function of time if the change in length gradually occurs over a 60 millisecond interval. (The change in length is effected by the speaker's lips and larynx.)

5.   During the production of the sound discussed in exercise 4, the fundamental frequency of phonation changed from 100 Hz to 250 Hz. Sketch the fundamental frequency of phonation and the first two harmonics if this change occurred in a linear manner. Are the graphs of the formant frequencies and fundamental frequency and its harmonics similar? Why?

5

Speech analysis

Instrumental analysis is necessary to understand how vocal communication works. Auditory transcriptions of speech can never isolate the acoustic cues that specify the sounds of speech. We can, for example, listen to as many carefully transcribed tokens of the syllables [di] and [du] as we care to, without ever discovering that different acoustic cues specify the "identical" sound [d] in these two syllables. As listeners, we have no more direct knowledge of the process of speech perception than we, as eaters of ice-cream, have of the enzyme systems that are involved in the digestion of sugar. If we want to study the digestion of sugar we have to make use of instrumental techniques. Likewise we have to make use of instrumental techniques for the analysis of speech.

In this chapter we will discuss both recent computer-implemented techniques and the sound spectrograph. The sound spectrograph was the instrument of choice for the analysis of speech from 1940 through the 1970s when computer-implemented methods began to be substituted. Computer-implemented techniques are now usually more accurate and can derive data that the sound spectrograph inherently cannot. However, the distinction between computer-implemented procedures and the sound spectrograph is beginning to blur; recent "digital" versions of the sound spectrograph are really dedicated microprocessors. Nevertheless, the sound spectrograph in either its traditional analog version or recent digital versions is often better suited for certain tasks, for example, showing formant frequency transitions, monitoring the speech samples of subjects, and tracking the acoustic changes consequent to rapid articulatory movements during physiological experiments, etc.

Both the capabilities and the limitations of the sound spectrograph must be understood in order to interpret the data of the many studies that relied on this instrument. We will also briefly discuss techniques for tape recording that minimize distortion, and review current computer-analysis techniques that can be applied in the acoustic analysis of speech.

The sound spectrograph

The sound spectrograph was probably the single most useful device for the quantitative analysis of speech. The sound spectrograph was developed at Bell Telephone Laboratories in connection with work on analysis–synthesis speech transmission systems like the Vocoder, which we will discuss in Chapter 7. The sound spectrograph can be used to make various types of analyses of acoustic signals; we will discuss the most useful applications for speech analysis. Detailed discussions of the circuitry of the machine and other applications can be found in Koenig, Dunn and Lacey (1946), Potter, Kopp and Green (1947), and Flanagan (1972).

The output that the machine yields is a piece of paper called a *spectrogram*. There have been attempts to use spectrograms to identify people's voices. The promoters of these endeavors have applied the term *voiceprint* to the spectrogram (Kersta, 1962). The term "voiceprint," of course, brings to mind the term "fingerprint." However, research results suggest that it is far from clear that people can be identified through the use of spectrograms with the certainty of fingerprints (Bolt *et al.*, 1973; Tosi *et al.*, 1972). There have been several independent attempts to develop the use of sound spectrograms for voice identification. For example, the central project of the scientists imprisoned in the Soviet slave labor camp in Alexander Solzhenitsyn's novel, *The First Circle*, is the development of a voice identification device.

The sound spectrograph essentially performs two sequential operations. The first step in an analysis is to record a speech signal on the machine. The usual "input" is from a magnetic tape recorder, because the first step of a real analysis is to record the speech signals of interest. We will discuss later in this chapter some of the precautions that one should take when making tape recordings. The *speech input* is thus usually from a tape recorder playing a previously recorded signal. The sound spectrograph machines that are commercially available, for example some models of the Kay Elemetrics Corporation, have a number of input channels, which are controlled by a switch. You can thus connect either a tape recorder or a microphone to the machine and select the input that you want. Traditional analog versions of the sound spectrograph record the input signal on a magnetic medium that goes around the outside edge of a thin drum or disk. The recording head, which is similar to the recording head on a conventional tape recorder, forms a magnetic "image" on the edge of the magnetic recording disk when the sound spectrograph is switched into its "record" mode. Recent digital versions of the sound spectrograph convert the input signal into a digital representation which is stored in an electronic memory.

Functionally there is little difference between the basic analysis performed by digital or analog versions of the sound spectrograph. The duration of the segment that can be analyzed in one pass by the Kay Elemetrics digital sound spectrograph is longer than the analog sound spectrograph, 5 seconds compared to 2 seconds and additional analyses can be carried out with greater precision and reliability. The digital sound spectrographs of other companies record signals that have different durations and have somewhat different modes of analysis. However, the basic principles are similar for all sound spectrographs. The discussion of the sound spectrograph that follows will focus on the traditional analog version that is still found in many laboratories, and that was the source of most quantitative data for studies published through the mid 1970s.

The recording head converts the electrical signal that corresponds to the speech signal into a magnetic field that is impressed on the magnetic recording medium. This is, of course, similar to the process that is the basis of practically all magnetic tape recorders. As is the case in a conventional tape recorder, the "level" of the input signal must be kept within a range appropriate for the machine and recording medium. If the electrical signal that is being recorded is too large, the magnetic image is likely to be distorted. If the electrical signal is too small the magnetic image will not be discernible when it is reproduced. The situation is no different for digital versions of the sound spectrograph. If the input signal is recorded at too high a level, it will be distorted. If it is recorded at too low a level, it will not provide an adequate signal-to-noise ratio for analysis. The *record level* thus has to be kept within certain limits. This is not very difficult because there is a meter or digital readout on the machine and a "record level adjustment" knob. You simply set the record level to the value specified in the machine's instructions. The problem is similar to setting the brightness control on a television set. If the control is set at too high a value, the image on the television set will be "washed out"; if it is too low you will be unable to see the image. The sound spectrograph level setting problem is in some ways simpler than setting the brightness level of a television set because you have a calibrated meter on the sound spectrograph. Most tape recorders have level meters or level-indicating devices. These meters or devices take into account the acoustic properties of human speech and the recording electrical and magnetic properties of the recorder, and good recordings of speech signals can be made by keeping the level at or slightly under the value specified in the instructions. As in interstate driving, you have to keep *under* a maximum and *over* a minimum "limit."

There are, however, some important differences between recording an input signal on a sound spectrograph and on a conventional tape recorder. The most obvious difference is that the conventional analog spectrograph will only record a 2.2 second sample of speech. If the spectrograph is left in its "record" function, it will record a new message signal, erasing the material that was previously recorded on it, as the magnetic disk rotates past the recording head. The proper technique in using the spectrograph is thus to set the machine into its "record" function, record a 2 second sample of speech, and then immediately switch the machine from its "record" to its "reproduce" function. If you have set the correct record level on the meter you will then have a 2 second sample recorded on the magnetic disk. The spectrograph has a monitor loudspeaker so it is possible to listen and to verify that you have recorded the appropriate material. It is easy to set the appropriate record level when a tape recording is the speech input source. If the level is not correct you can adjust the record level control, stop the tape recorder, rewind, and play it back again.

The meter that is used to adjust the record level is adjusted to yield a good recording when the *peak* signal does not exceed 0 VU. The VU scale is an old method of measuring sound levels that originated in the days of radio network AM broadcasts. The dimensional term *VU* signifies "volume units" and the meter is designed to respond to speech signals in a manner that will produce deflections of the meter's needle that are easy to follow when the input to the meter is a speech signal. It is easy to make tape recordings or sound spectrograms that are distorted when the VU meter readings of "odd" signals like bird calls are interpreted as though they were human speech signals. Computer-implemented analysis techniques, which Greenewalt (1968) first used, are better suited for the analysis of birdsong.

There is one additional control on the spectrograph which is specially adapted for the analysis of speech signals. The spectrograph has an *input shaping* control which can be set to either a "flat" or "HS" (high frequency shaping) position. The "HS" position is usually used when speech signals are being analyzed. It switches in an electrical network that emphasizes the high frequencies of the speech signal. As we noted in Chapter 4, the amplitude of the glottal source falls off at the rate of 6 dB per octave. This means that there is less energy in the acoustic speech signal at higher frequencies. The HS circuits compensate for this decrease in energy and compensate in part for the limited ability of the spectrograph to indicate a wide range of amplitudes. Amplitude is indicated by the darkness of the images on the paper; the paper has a very limited dark-to-light dynamic range. These circuits are used whenever the machine is being used to make normal spectrograms of adult humans. The "flat" setting is sometimes useful for the analysis of the speech of infants, who have proportionately more energy at high frequencies, or for the analysis of nonspeech signals. It is also useful for making spectrograph "sections," which we will discuss later.

The way in which the spectrograph performs an analysis may be clearer if we first consider a simpler form of frequency analysis. Suppose that someone

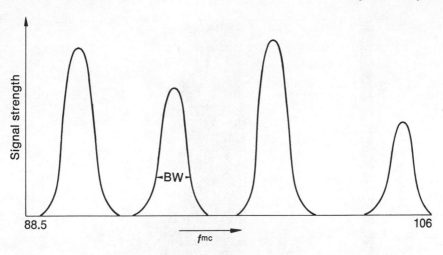

Figure 5.1. A plot of signal strength of FM radio stations. BW refers to bandwidth.

asked you to provide a graph that showed the frequencies at which FM radio stations were broadcasting in Providence, Rhode Island, at or about 12 noon on December 10 and the relative amplitude of each station's broadcast as received in your home. The request would be very easy to satisfy if you had a radio receiver that had a "tuning meter" that measured signal strength. The "tuning control" on a radio is a control that adjusts the frequency of a variable electronic filter. As you adjust the tuning control, the filter lets electromagnetic energy within a certain range of frequencies through into a series of amplifiers and other devices that ultimately produce an audible signal. The variable electronic filter that you "set" to "select" the appropriate radio station has a fixed bandwidth and an adjustable center frequency. When the tuning control is set to 88.5 the electronic filter's center frequency is 88.5×10 Hz. When the dial is moved to 100, its center frequency is 100×10 Hz, etc. If you systematically tuned to each station in Providence and wrote down the "signal strength" that the radio's meter noted, you would be able to make the graph that appears in Figure 5.1. The signal strength meter of the radio (probably only a relatively expensive "high fidelity" tuner would have this type of meter) measures the amplitude of the received signal; this is plotted on the vertical scale. The horizontal scale represents the settings of the tuner's dial. Note that there is a range of frequencies for each radio station that corresponds, in part, to the bandwidth of the tuner's filter. The bandwidth of the tuner's filter also roughly matches the band of frequencies that each station broadcasts.

The graph of Figure 5.1 is a sort of spectrum of the FM broadcast frequencies in a particular location at a particular time. It was made by taking a single variable filter and moving it through the frequency range of interest and

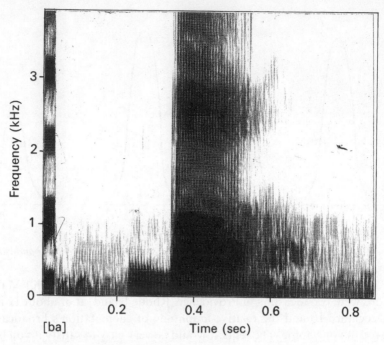

Figure 5.2. Wide-band spectrogram of the sound [ba].

keeping track of the amplitude of the signal at each setting of the variable filter. The sound spectrograph operates in essentially the same manner. Displays that are similar, in principle, to that of Figure 5.1 can be made for a speech signal for a particular interval of time. These displays are called *sections*. The usual spectrograph display provides information on the intensity of energy in the speech signal as a function of both frequency and time over the full 2.2 second interval recorded on the spectrograph's magnetic disk for the analog machine.

A spectrogram of the syllable [ba] uttered by an adult male speaker of American English is shown in Figure 5.2. The vertical scale is a frequency scale. Note that it is a *linear* scale, i.e. a given interval of frequency is equivalent to a fixed interval throughout the frequency scale. The spectrograph can be set to make spectrograms with either a linear or a logarithmic scale. The linear scale is best if one wants to make quantitative measurements from the spectrogram. Note that the frequency scale runs from 0 to 4 kHz. The spectrograph was equipped with a "scale expander" unit that allows one to match the vertical scale of the spectrogram to the frequency range of interest. The formant frequencies of interest of the sounds on the spectrogram all fall below 4 kHz so the freqency scale was "expanded' to cover the range 0–4 kHz. If the "scale expander" had not been used, the vertical scale would have encompassed the range 0–8 kHz, but the upper half of the spectrogram would not have contained any useful information and we would have half the detail in the 0–4 kHz range, where the useful acoustic material is displayed. Note also the short, straight "bars" that occur at 1, 2, 3, and 4 kHz near the vertical scale. These bars are frequency calibrating signals that can be placed on the spectrogram. Their use is strongly recommended since they reduce the likelihood of measurement errors.

The dark "bands" of the sound [ba] indicate the presence of local energy peaks in the spectrum of these sounds as functions of time. In other words, there are local peaks at about 700 Hz, 1100 Hz, and 2800 Hz at 0.4 second. There is also a very low frequency peak at about 140 Hz. The dark bands at 700 Hz, 1100 Hz, and 2800 Hz are the spectrogram's response to the formant frequencies of the vowel [a]. The dark band at 140 Hz reflects the fundamental frequency of phonation. The fundamental frequency can be determined more accurately by counting the number of vertical striations that appear in the dark bands per unit of time. Note that all the dark bands actually consist of vertical striations. This spectrogram is a "wide-band" analysis that was made using the 300 Hz bandwidth analyzing filter of the spectrograph apparatus. The 300 Hz bandwidth filter obviously does not have a good frequency resolution. You can see this in the width of the bands that correspond to the frequency calibrations of the spectrograph machine. The bands are about 300 Hz wide although the calibration signals actually consist of "pure" sinusoids, i.e. single frequencies. The wide-bandwidth analyzing filter, however, responds rapidly to changes in the energy of the acoustic signal. It therefore shows the fluctuations in the energy of the speech signal that occur as the vocal tract is excited by the glottal output.

In the spectrogram in Figure 5.2 you can see that the spacing between these striations varies in the course of time. In the interval between 0.35 and 0.45 second, 14 striations occur. The average fundamental period in that interval is 0.07 second, i.e. 70 milliseconds. The "average" fundamental frequency for this interval of speech is therefore equal to 140 Hz. The calculations that lead to this result are quite simple. Since 14 striations occur in 100 milliseconds the average period must be equal to

$$T = \frac{100}{14} = 7.14 \text{ msec}$$

If we recall the definition of fundamental frequency from Chapter 3,

$$f_0 = \frac{1}{T} = \frac{1}{7.14 \text{ msec}} = \frac{1}{0.00714} = 140 \text{ Hz}$$

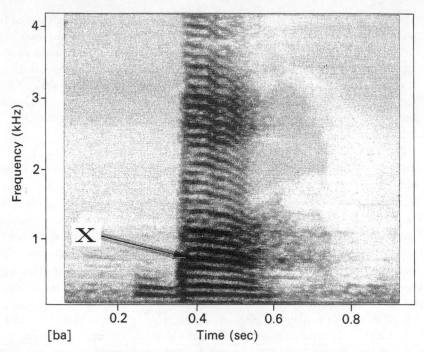

Figure 5.3. Narrow-band spectrogram of the same sound [ba] analyzed in Figure 5.2. The symbol X denotes the fifth harmonic of the fundamental frequency.

A "narrow-band" spectrogram of the same utterance is shown in Figure 5.3. Note the different appearance of this spectrogram. The only difference in the analysis is the substitution of a 50 Hz bandwidth analyzing filter. The dark "bands" of this spectrogram now reflect the energy that is present in the fundamental frequency and each harmonic of the glottal excitation. By measuring the frequency of the first harmonic, we can determine that the fundamental frequency is 140 Hz at $t = 0.4$ second. It is easier to "read" the value of the fundamental frequency by looking at the fifth harmonic, which is marked by an X in this figure. The frequency of this harmonic is by definition equal to $5f_0$. If you wanted to derive the fundamental frequency of phonation for this syllable as a function of time you could mark the fifth harmonic on the spectrogram and then trace it through the syllable. If you transferred the time scale and remembered to divide the vertical frequency scale by 5, you would have a plot of the fundamental frequency.

You would gain two advantages by tracing the fifth harmonic: (1) it is easier to measure than the fundamental frequency, and (2) variations in fundamental frequency are "magnified" five times. If the fundamental frequency fell 10 Hz, for example, the fifth harmonic would fall 50 Hz. It would be almost impossible to see a 10 Hz variation on the spectrogram; the 50 Hz fall is easy to see. Note in Figure 5.3 that the fundamental frequency falls rapidly in the interval between $t = 0.5$ second and $t = 0.6$ second. The change can be seen most clearly by tracing the change in frequency of the fifth harmonic. Still higher harmonics can be traced for more detail. The limit arises from the decreasing energy in the higher harmonics, which is a characteristic of the glottal source. However, the spectrogram may not always mark the higher harmonics.

The narrow-band filter also does not respond to rapid changes in the fundamental frequency. At the end of phonation there are typically a few long glottal periods that have less energy in their higher harmonics. These transients occur because the speaker is opening his vocal cords at the end of phonation and also lowering his pulmonary air pressure (Lieberman, 1967). We will discuss the mechanisms that regulate fundamental frequency in detail in Chapter 6, but you can see these transient conditions in the wide-band spectrogram in Figure 5.2. Note the longer spacing of the "voicing" striations, which reflects the long glottal periods, and the absence of darkening at higher frequencies in the wide-band spectrogram at the end of the syllable.

Interpreting spectrograms – how the spectrograph works

Comparing Figures 5.2 and 5.3, you can see a large difference between the appearance of the two spectrograms. It is essential to know why these two displays of the same signal look so different; this entails knowing how the spectrograph apparatus works. If you do not know how the spectrograph makes these displays, you can easily misinterpret sound spectrograms. Spectrograms are always difficult to interpret, but you can make absurd errors if you do not know what the machine is doing. This does not mean that you have to be a graduate electrical engineer and know the electronics of the sound spectrograph, but simply that you understand the general principles of the machine. If you know how the spectrograph works, you can avoid introducing artifacts into your data. You can also learn how to circumvent some of its limitations.

In Figure 5.4 the functional elements of a hypothetical "photo-output" narrow-band spectrograph machine have been sketched. The variable analyzing filter has a 50 Hz bandwidth, and its center frequency can be shifted to cover the frequency range between 0 and 8 kHz. The filter feeds into an amplifier and then into an averaging device, which removes small fluctuations in the filter's output. The averaged output, in turn, goes into a small light bulb. The brightness of the light bulb thus is a function of the electrical current from the filter. If the filter responds to a peak in the acoustic spectrum, the light bulb

59

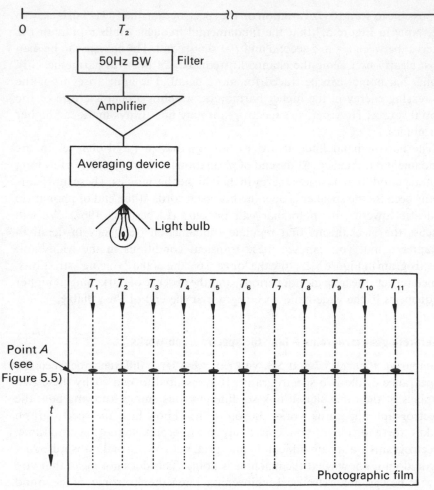

Figure 5.4. Sketch of a hypothetical "photo-output" narrow-band sound spectrograph machine.

will burn brighter. A low-level acoustic signal will result in a slight glow, an intermediate acoustic level in an intermediate brightness, etc. If the light bulb's output were focused on a photographic film, the film after development would be darker for a high acoustic level and lighter when the acoustic level was lower. The darkness of the film would reflect the level of the acoustic signal within the range of frequencies that the variable input filter was "set" to cover. If we provided a suitable mechanical system we could pull a piece of film past on a "track" T_1 while the filter that was set to a particular frequency range "scanned" a speech signal. The density of the film along that track would correspond to the presence of acoustic energy within that range of frequencies as a function of time. If we then adjusted the frequency range of the variable filter to a higher range of frequencies, moved the light bulb to track T_2, and repeated the process with the same speech sample, we would record a second track of variable density on the film.

The traditional sound spectrograph is functionally very similar to this photo-output spectrograph. The acoustic signal is recorded on the magnetic disk, which also holds a piece of special paper. The paper is darkened by the current that flows through the wire stylus of the spectrograph. The current that flows through the stylus is a function of the acoustic energy that the spectrograph's variable filter admits. As the spectrograph's disk turns round and round in its "analysis" mode, a mechanical system adjusts the range of frequencies that the variable filter admits, while it simultaneously moves the stylus up the sensitized paper. The darkening of the spectrogram paper at a particular location thus shows when the filter has admitted acoustic energy at a particular frequency range at some particular point in time. Recent digital versions of the sound spectrograph have substituted electronic circuits for mechanical devices but they are functionally similar and do the same job. The sound spectrograph does not have the dynamic range of a photographic film. This means that the range of dark-to-light gradations on the spectrogram cannot encompass the range of intensity that actually occurs in a real speech signal. The sound spectrograph therefore makes use of additional electronic processing to compensate for this deficiency.

In Figure 5.5 part of the spectrum of the sound [ə], which was shown in Figure 4.4, is shown at the top of the diagram. The plot beneath it is a hypothetical plot of the light output that might be measured for our photo-output spectrograph as a function of frequency at a particular point in time. This would be a "section" of the signal at point A in Figure 5.4. The "width" of each of the bars on the light-output graph is, of course, 50 Hz because of the bandwidth of the spectrograph's analyzing filter. The vertical height of these bars would correspond to the density of the developed film on our hypothetical photo-output spectrograph. However, we have noted that we cannot handle this range of density with the paper that is used on the actual spectrograph machine. The spectrograph machine solves this problem by a two-stage process. The amplitude range of the output of the analyzing filter is first "compressed" by an "automatic gain control" (AGC) system. This is equivalent to a little man sitting inside the machine who rapidly turns a volume control, "turning up" the lower level signals and "turning down" the high level signals. The spectrograph machine thus has a control labeled "AGC" which controls the degree to which this adjustment is carried out. In Figure 5.5 the third graph shows this output with a moderate amount of AGC action. There

61

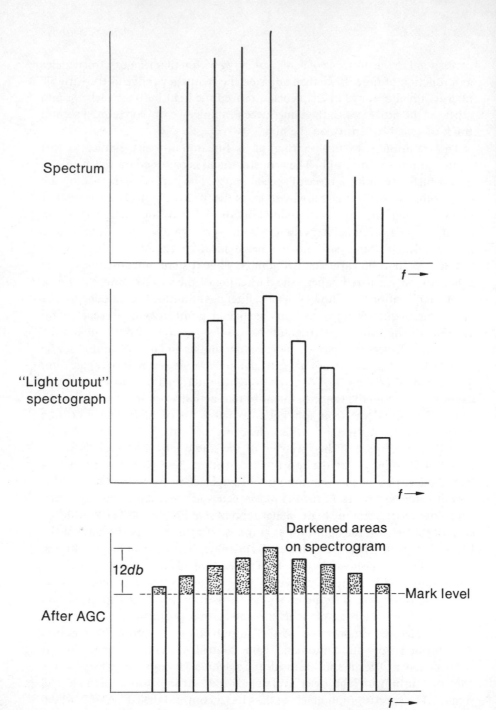

Figure 5.5. Spectrum of a speech signal and two stages of processing in the spectrograph machine.

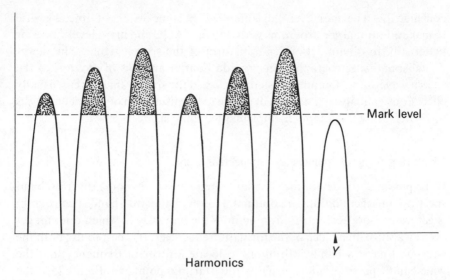

Figure 5.6. The effect of "mark level" on a spectrogram. Note that the machine would not darken the spectrogram at harmonic Y although acoustic energy is actually present there.

still are differences between the amplitudes of different harmonics but they are reduced. The range of densities that the spectrograph paper can handle is about 12 dB. The setting of the "mark level" control on the spectrograph machine, which is indicated by the dashed line that goes across the third graph in Figure 5.5, shows this control set to produce a spectrogram in which the relative amplitude of each harmonic of the spectrum is portrayed on the spectrogram *after* AGC action. Amplitudes less than the value of the dashed line will not be marked at all; levels above it will be proportionately darker.

It is obvious that the darkness of any "bar" on the spectrogram is affected by the settings of the AGC and the mark level controls. If the mark level control were set to the level shown in Figure 5.6 the spectrogram would not "show" any energy present at harmonic *Y* although, in fact, energy was present there. The interpretation of a spectrogram is, on this count alone, a difficult undertaking since what you see depends on the setting of the AGC and mark level controls. Some spectrograph machines do not offer a choice of AGC and mark level settings, but the problem still remains. The only difference is that the manufacturer has set the controls inside the machine. It is sometimes tempting to conclude that there is no energy at some harmonic of the fundamental because no line appears on a particular spectrogram at the expected frequency. This conclusion might not be warranted; it might be an artifact of the settings of the AGC and mark level values. Before one can

63

conclude that a harmonic has "disappeared" at some instant of time, it is wise to make additional spectrograms with different AGC and mark level values or better still, to obtain a Fourier transform of the speech signal. The newer digital sound spectrographs can provide Fourier analysis of sections of the speech waveform. Computer systems designed for speech analysis can usually effect Fourier analyses, and we will return to the discussion of Fourier analysis in connection with computer-implemented analysis.

Measuring formant frequencies on spectrograms

It is possible to determine formant frequencies in some narrow-band spectrograms if conditions are optimal. However, the wide-band spectrogram is generally more accurate and sometimes the only way in which one can get even an approximate idea of the formant frequencies. It is best to use both the wide- and narrow-bandwidth filters to locate a formant frequency, but the wide-band spectrogram is usually the starting point. In Figure 5.7 the spectrum of the [ə] sound (cf. Figure 4.4) is again displayed. The fundamental frequency of phonation is 100 Hz, and harmonics thus occur at 100 Hz intervals. The analyzing bandwidth of the 300 Hz bandwidth filter is shown schematically as the filter just begins to admit the acoustic energy at the fundamental frequency in block 1. The averaged output of the filter is sketched below it. Note that the output of the filter will continue to rise as it moves upwards in frequency from block 1 to block 2 to block 3, because the filter will admit additional harmonics of the speech signal. The filter's output will continue to increase as its center frequency (cf. Chapter 3) moves upwards in frequency until it is at 500 Hz. There is no point at which the filter's output is zero, because the filter's bandwidth is so wide (i.e. 300 Hz) that it is always admitting at least three harmonics once its center frequency is past 150 Hz. As the amplitude of the harmonics falls after 500 Hz, the filter's output also falls. The output of the filter approximates the "envelope" of the spectrum of the sound [ə]. (The "envelope" is the function that connects the peak of each harmonic with the peak of the adjacent harmonic.)

If appropriate AGC and mark level settings are used on the spectrograph apparatus, the final spectrogram will have darkened "bars" at the three peaks that are shaded in the graph of the filter output in Figure 5.7. The wide-band spectrogram thus provides information on the local peaks in the spectrum's "envelope," which reflects, in part, the formant frequencies of the sound.

The wide-band spectrogram will "show" the approximate location of a formant even when there is no energy present at the actual formant frequency *if* the fundamental frequency is at least half the bandwidth of the analyzing filter. In Figure 5.8 the low frequency end of the spectrum of an [i] sound (the vowel

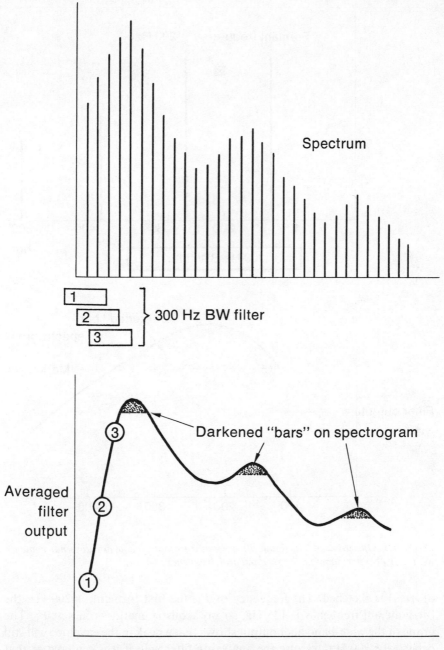

Figure 5.7. Functional operation of wide-band filtering of spectrograph. The input spectrum is averaged by the wide-band filter and the formant frequencies appear as darkened bars on the spectrogram.

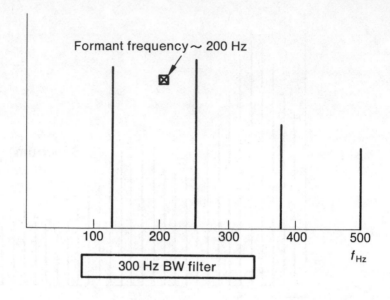

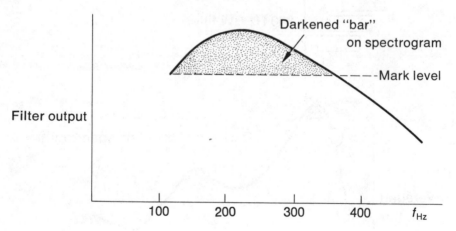

Figure 5.8. Operation of wide-band filter when a formant frequency does not coincide with that of a harmonic of the fundamental frequency.

of *meet*) is sketched. The frequency of F_1, the first formant, is 200 Hz; the fundamental frequency is 125 Hz, so no acoustic energy occurs at F_1. The graph of the wide-band filter output shows that a peak in the envelope will still occur near 200 Hz, because the analyzing filter will, if it is centered at that frequency, pass the two harmonics at 125 and 250 Hz. These two harmonics have the greatest amplitudes, so the peak in the filter output function will be centered at approximately 200 Hz. The darkened area on the spectrogram will, of course, be about 300 Hz wide, but it will be centered on the formant frequency. Note that a narrow-band spectrogram would *not* show the formant frequencies. It would introduce an additional source of error into the measurement of the formant frequency because it would produce dark bars at the harmonics. We might be able to see that the harmonic at 250 Hz was darker than at 125 and 375Hz. Thus, the harmonic would indicate that the formant frequency was near 250 Hz, but we would not be able to tell that it was at 200 Hz. The frequency resolution of the narrow-band spectrogram is greater than that of the wide-band spectrogram, but it does not necessarily yield greater precision in the measurement of formant frequencies. This follows from the point that we stressed in Chapter 4, that the formant frequencies are properties of the filter function of the supralaryngeal vocal tract. *The formant frequencies are the frequencies at which the supralaryngeal filter would let maximum acoustic energy through.* The electronic processing of the sound spectrograph is a means whereby we can often derive useful information that can help us locate formant frequencies. It does not directly "show" formant frequencies.

Variations in the settings of the AGC and mark level controls of the spectrograph apparatus can also produce wide-band spectrograms of the same acoustic signal that look very different, and we cannot assume that a formant frequency has "disappeared" because it is not marked. We likewise have to be very careful to avoid interpreting every dark bar as though it reflects the presence of a formant frequency. The fundamental frequency of phonation of normal adult male human beings often exceeds 200 Hz during connected discourse. Normal adult females usually have average fundamental frequencies in excess of 200 Hz. In Figure 5.9 the uppermost spectrogram is a wide-band spectrogram made by using the usual 300 Hz bandwidth setting. The sound that is being analyzed is the word *bad*, transcribed [bæd]. Note the wide bars on the spectrogram that are spaced apart at intervals of 250–300 Hz. Do these bars show the formant frequency variation of this sound? Should we rush to our typewriter and send off a communication to a scholarly journal announcing the "discovery" of a sound that has at least ten formant frequencies between 250 Hz and 3000 Hz?

The answer to this question is, of course, No! The narrow-band, 50 Hz bandwidth spectrogram of this same utterance, which appears in Figure 5.9B, shows the same set of darkened bars. The width of the bars made with the 50 Hz bandwidth analyzing filter is less, and the bars do not show some of the variations that are evident in the spectrogram of Figure 5.9A, but the dark bands of both spectrograms primarily reflect the *harmonic* structure of the glottal source. The fundamental frequency of the utterance exceeds 250 Hz and is so high that the 300 Hz bandwidth filter can not "take in" at least two

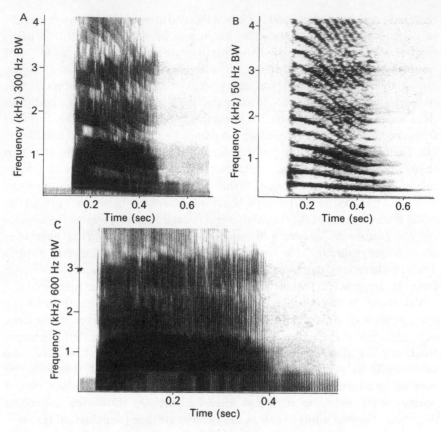

Figure 5.9. The spectrographic analysis of a speaker whose fundamental frequency exceeds 200 Hz. (A) 300 Hz bandwidth spectrogram. (B) 50 Hz bandwidth spectrogram. (C) 600 Hz bandwidth spectrogram.

harmonics. The output of the analyzing filter thus is *not* a measure of the envelope of the spectrum and the dark bands on the spectrogram do not manifest the formant frequencies.

We can increase the bandwidth of the spectrograph's analyzing filter by a simple artifice. If we present the speech signal to the analyzing filter at half speed, we will divide all the frequencies on the recording by one-half. The fundamental frequency of phonation now becomes 125 Hz, and the 300 Hz bandwidth analyzing filter can now take two harmonics. The lowest spectrogram shows the half-speed analysis. The formant structure of the utterance is now evident. Note that the formant frequency pattern at the end of the utterance does not match the fundamental frequency variation. The formant frequencies do not fall in the interval between 0.2 and 0.4 second, whereas the fundamental frequency does in spectrograms A and B. Note that the time scale of the bottom spectrogram is expanded compared to the scale for the two spectrograms made at normal speed. The effective bandwidth of the spectrograph's wide-band analyzing filter is 600 Hz when we make a spectrogram at half speed.

It is simple to make half-speed spectrograms with the traditional Kay spectrograph by recording with the recording speed selector set at the position labeled 16 000 Hz. The same effect can be achieved by re-recording the tape to a speed that is twice the playback speed on those sound spectrographs that analyze the signal directly from a "loop" of a tape recording. The scale expander unit is very useful when you do this because the frequency scale can be adjusted to a useful range. (The half-speed spectrogram that appears in Figure 5.9 was made with scale expander set to 25 percent to get a vertical scale of 4000 Hz).

It is important to remember that the dark bars on wide-band spectrograms often simply manifest the harmonics of the fundamental frequency. The range of fundamental frequency variation in normal speech often usually exceeds one octave and sometimes reaches two octaves. An adult male speaker whose "average" fundamental frequency is 100 Hz will usually reach at least 200 Hz in connected speech. The fundamental frequency variations may not be perceived as being especially high because they are not sustained, but they will show up in the spectrogram. The "staircase" effect that you can see in the spectrogram in Figure 5.10 at $t = 1.0$ second occurs when the fundamental frequency is at the point of being too high for the spectrograph to derive the envelope of the spectrum. The dark areas at $t = 0.2$ second reflect the formant frequencies of the vowel [ə] but the bars then also begin to track the individual harmonics.

The formant frequencies of the utterances of speakers who have extremely high fundamental frequencies can often be more readily determined by selecting for analysis an utterance that is "breathy", i.e. whispered, or produced with mixed noise and phonation. The spectrum of a noise source has energy throughout a range of frequencies rather than at discrete, harmonically related frequencies as is the case for the glottal source during phonation. Energy is present at all frequencies within the range that characterizes the noise source, so the analyzing filter of the spectrograph can derive the spectrum envelope during the breathy part of an utterance. In Figure 5.11 a breathy utterance of a newborn infant is shown. The formant frequencies are evident at 1.1, 3.3, and 5.0 kHz. The fundamental frequency of phonation is about 400 Hz. If the cry did not have a breathy, noisy quality (i.e. noise mixed with phonation), it would not have been possible to measure the formant frequencies in this way.

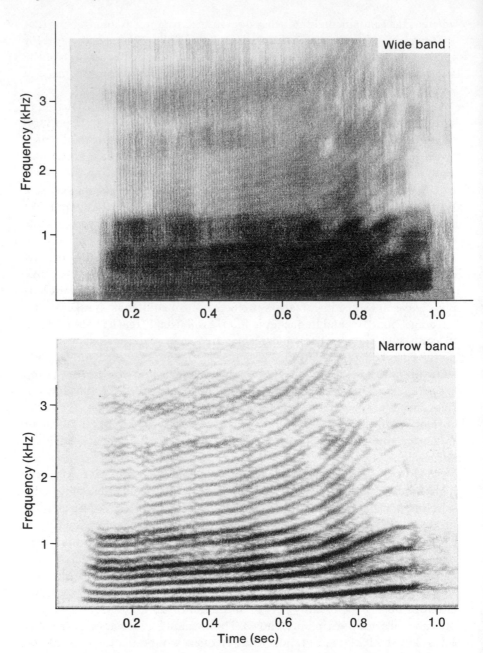

Figure 5.10. Note the "staircase" effect on the wide-band spectrogram. The fundamental frequency is at the point of being too high for the spectrograph to resolve the formant frequencies.

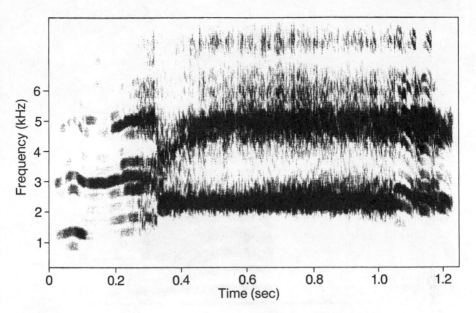

Figure 5.11. Spectrogram of breathy utterance of a newborn infant. The "noise" excitation makes it possible to resolve the formant frequencies although the fundamental frequency is very high.

If the AGC and mark level controls of the spectrograph are carefully adjusted, it is possible to determine the approximate locations of formants for voices that have high fundamental frequencies. This is done by looking at the relative darkness of the harmonics. In Figure 5.12 the formant frequencies of the sound are near 500, 1200, and 2500 Hz. There is obviously a great deal of inherent uncertainty here because we do not have acoustic information at intervals closer than 300 Hz, which is the fundamental frequency of phonation for this utterance. The spectrographic "section" which would show the relative amplitude of each harmonic for a sample of time of 100 milliseconds would not really provide much more information. Energy still would be present at intervals of 300 Hz. As we noted in Chapter 4, human beings have no difficulty in deriving the formant frequencies of sounds like this.

The different analyzing filter bandwidths and sectioning devices of the spectrograph can all be used together to determine the formant frequencies of sounds like the vowel [a], where two formants are close in frequency. It is easier to determine these formant frequencies if you have wide-band and narrow-band displays. Computer-implemented analysis is better still, but the combination of the wide-band and the narrow-band spectrogram is often sufficient to determine the formant frequencies with reasonable accuracy. As we have noted, there are definite limits on the precision that is necessary to specify the formant frequencies.

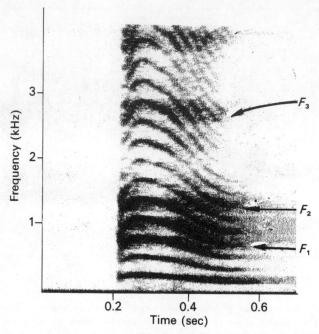

Figure 5.12. Using a narrow-band, 50 Hz bandwidth spectrogram to estimate formant frequencies.

Some precautions and techniques for measuring formant frequencies

In Figure 5.13 a line is traced through the center of the dark bands that reflect F_1, F_2, and F_3 in the spectrogram. It is useful to trace the presumed position of each formant directly on the spectrogram with a pencil line before you attempt to measure the frequency value. If you make a mistake or arrive at an odd result later you then can work back through the measurement process step by step. If you were to measure the formant frequency from the spectrogram by means of a calibrated scale without marking the spectrogram, you might not be able to trace the point at which you were in error. Note that the "zero" frequency line in the spectrogram has some dark traces beneath it. These traces are a mirror image of the display above the zero line. The spectrograph can be adjusted to eliminate this "mirror image" effect, but it is safer to set the zero frequency line for each spectrogram by means of the mirror image. The spectrograph's electronic circuits tend to change their properties with time as they "warm up." If you do not use the mirror image technique, it is possible to introduce systematic errors as the zero line drifts to some new unknown nonzero value.

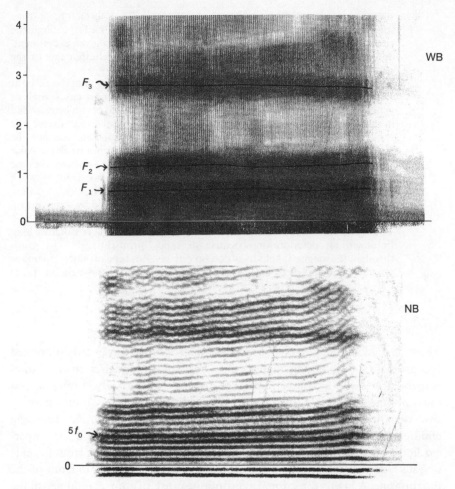

Figure 5.13. Using the mirror image technique for "zero" frequency calibration. The formant frequencies are noted on the upper wide-band spectrogram. The fifth harmonic of the fundamental frequency is marked on the lower narrow-band spectrogram.

Tape recording techniques

The precautions that are generally relevant for tape recording apply with special force when recording speech signals for analysis. Three criteria must be kept in mind.

(1)   Speech signals must be recorded without distortion, i.e. the recorded signal must be an accurate representation of the acoustic signal. Nevertheless, the frequency and dynamic range recorded do not usually have to meet the

73

standards for "high fidelity" recordings of music. They instead have to be sufficient to describe accurately the acoustic correlates of the linguistic contrasts or emotional affects that are being analyzed in a given experiment, and they have to be sufficiently accurate to meet the requirements of the particular analysis procedure being used.

(2) The signal-to-noise ratio should be maximized. That is, the signal should be at least 20 dB above the level of background noise. In most cases analysis procedures will not work unless the voice of a single speaker can be recorded in a quiet environment. For example, pitch extractors that derive the fundamental frequency of phonation need a recorded signal that contains the speech signal of only one speaker. The pitch extractor cannot track the voice of one speaker when a second voice simultaneously occurs, as is often the case when one records a normal conversation. Nor will pitch extractors work when competing periodic noises occur, for example, when the tape recording contains the low frequency, low amplitude sounds produced by some central air-conditioning systems.

(3) The signal should be recorded so that it can be stored for a reasonably long time without deteriorating because of tape "print-through". In print-through, the magnetic field recorded on one layer of tape produces an image on adjacent layers of tape. Listening to a tape with print-through, one hears the signal echoing in the background.

Microphones

The wide availability of electret condensor microphones has greatly simplified the problem of obtaining high quality recordings. Electret microphones respond directly to the sound pressure of the speech signal. Directional electret microphones can be obtained that respond differentially to sounds coming from one direction. This can be an advantage if one is, for example, recording children in their home environment. A highly directional "cardiod" or "super-cardiod" microphone in effect, does not "hear" sounds coming from the side or back and will enhance the recording of the person directly in front of the microphone. A highly directional microphone must, of course, be aimed at the subject. It will not necessarily pick up the mother's voice without attenuation on when it is aimed at the child, unless the mother is positioned near the child.

The choice of microphone will depend on the goal of a particular research project. Electret microphones can be purchased that are relatively inexpensive. These microphones will suffice for studies in which one simply wants to determine the formant frequencies or fundamental frequency pattern of an utterance. Recording in a quiet environment, perhaps using a directional electret, is usually more important than using an expensive microphone. If the details of the onset spectrum and aspiration noise of stop consonants (cf. Chapters 7 and 8) are the focus of the research, quality electret or traditional condensor microphones and an echo-free acoustic environment will be necessary.

Tape recorders

Tape recorders likewise do not have to be laboratory-standard instruments for most studies. The frequency response of most reel-to-reel tape recorders is adequate for speech research at a recording speed of 7.5 inches per second. More expensive tape recorders usually have better signal-to-noise ratios, and more stability and accuracy in the speed at which they record. Cassette tape recorders generally have much lower signal-to-noise ratios than good reel-to-reel tape recorders. However, cassette recorders are practical instruments for many field studies. In this regard, the size and weight of a reel-to-reel tape recorder often has little relation to the quality of the recordings that it can produce. The Nagra portable tape recorders, for example, are smaller and lighter than most other reel-to-reel recorders but produce extremely high quality tape recordings. Nagra recorders unfortunately are also very expensive.

Any tape recorder can become misaligned so that the recording heads do not maintain proper contact with the tape. The frequency response and signal-to-noise ratio of a misaligned tape recorder will deteriorate. Magnetic heads can also become magnetized, lowering the signal-to-noise ratio. Apart from careful maintenance, in well-controlled studies it is essential to record known calibrating test signals on the tape recordings that will be analyzed. If a series of sinusoidal signals from a signal generator having constant amplitude is recorded on a tape recorder and subsequently analyzed using the spectrograph or computer system that will be used in the study, the total system (excluding the microphone) can be checked. Special microphone calibrators can be purchased when necessary.

Filters

The signal that is of interest in studies of speech is obviously the speech signal. In normal listening situations people adapt to and ignore low frequency ambient noises like the sounds produced by central air-conditioners. However, these pervasive low frequency ambient noises can interfere with or make acoustic analysis impossible. It thus is useful to use high-pass filters inserted as close to the input microphone as possible. Many high quality microphones (e.g. Shure, Sennheiser, and AKG microphones) have filters that will attenuate frequencies lower than 100 or 200 Hz. The filters are in many cases adjustable; different "cut-off" frequencies and filter slopes can be set. Tape recorders like the Nagra type 4.2, which is designed for field use, also have input filters that can be set to attenuate low frequency ambient noise.

Recording level and print-through

In making a tape recording that you intend to analyze, it is essential to avoid overmodulating the tape or recording the signal at too high a level. If you overmodulate the tape you will introduce electrical energy that, when analyzed, may look like acoustic energy. It may be impossible to differentiate the recording artifacts from the recorded acoustic signal. You can avoid these artifacts by not overmodulating the tape recording. The peaks registered during recording which indicate the amplitude of the signal should thus be kept below the red area that marks the overload region on many tape recorders.

You should also determine *what* the meter on your tape recorder is measuring. Less expensive or older recorders may have VU (volume unit) meters which show a frequency weighted average of the speech signal over an interval of about 100 milliseconds. The speech signal can have momentary peaks (for example, at the onset of stop consonants) that overload the tape recording, though the average registering on the VU meter is below the marked overload region. If one is analyzing the properties of bursts for stop consonants this can be a problem. It would be necessary to keep the recording level considerably lower than the marked, red overload region when using a tape recorder that had a simple VU meter. Tape recorders designed with acoustic analysis in mind, like the Nagra, have meters that lock onto the peaks in the speech signal; the speech signal can be recorded closer to the marked overload region using these metering systems.

In general, it is best to avoid recording a speech signal too near to the overload region. The speaker's voice may suddenly increase in loudness causing an overload until the operator manually lowers the system gain. AGC (automatic gain circuits) can be useful in certain instances, for example, where the analysis is not concerned with the characteristics of transient events. However, in general it is best to monitor the tape recording as it is being made, preferably by listening to the *recorded* signal using headphones on tape recorders where this is possible, and visually monitoring the metering device.

The use of a recording level that is low, but that still achieves a useful signal-to-noise ratio, is thus advisable. The signal-to-noise ratio that is necessary will depend on the analysis system and the particular procedure or computer algorithm to be used. The interactive computer-implemented speech analysis systems that are becoming available make it possible to specify the optimum recording level in particular instances. It is always appropriate to attempt the analysis of a trial recording using the equipment and computer programs that you intend to use for a complete study *before* you systematically record the entire test corpus. It is best to use as low a gain as possible to avoid the effects of overmodulation. The use of lower tape recording levels also helps to avoid the problem of tape print-through. It is advisable to use magnetic tape that is at least 1.0 mil (0.001 inch) thick to separate the layers of the magnetic medium on a reel of tape. Extra thick, 1.5 mil "low print-through" tape is still better.

Computer-implemented procedures

Although powerful digital computers have been available for many years, software and input–output devices suitable for the analysis of speech were available at only a few laboratories. These systems for computer-implemented analysis and synthesis of speech were designed for specific digital computer systems and research projects. The computer systems that had to be used were also fairly complex, expensive to buy, and expensive to maintain. The earliest systems were developed in the 1950s and were gradually perfected. Different research groups each developed different systems. However, these research projects were not carried out in complete isolation. An exchange of ideas occurred. The fruits of this long period of gradual development by different research groups are some basic procedures that have proved to be useful and that have been incorporated into almost every speech analysis–synthesis package.

More recently, software "packages" specifically designed for research on speech production and speech perception that can work on comparatively inexpensive computers are becoming readily available. These packages all differ and new products are continually being introduced that work on various computer systems. It would be difficult to describe the specific command structure of each different speech analysis program. It would be futile to try to anticipate programs that might become available. The discussion that follows will instead describe the "core" of basic procedures and the basic steps that all speech analysis programs incorporate. The discussion will also note some of the principles that underlie the synthesis of speech; the discussion of speech synthesis techniques will, however, be deferred to Chapter 7.

The basic components of a speech analysis system

The basic functional components that make up a computer-implemented speech analysis system involve:

(1)   Converting a continuous and thus analog speech signal into a digital representation that the computer programs can process. The system must also store these signals for analysis.

(2)   Displaying the stored speech samples so that relevant portions of the speech signal can be selected for analysis.

(3)   Performing time and frequency domain analyses and presenting the results of these analyses to the researcher.

Speech analysis

"Interactive" computer systems in which an individual looks at the waveforms and listens to the input and stored speech signals have been found to be most effective since they allow human intervention to correct and/or avoid artifacts. We will describe these basic operations in the remainder of this chapter. The illustrations of some of the details pertain to the BLISS system that has been developed at Brown University by John Mertus. This system is in use in a number of laboratories throughout the world and can be obtained from Brown University. However, the discussion will generally apply to other systems and speech analysis packages as well.

The input stage: analog-to-digital conversion

Quantization

Digital computer programs operate by means of mathematical algorithms that manipulate number sequences. The analog or continuous representation of the amplitude of the speech signal as a function of time must be converted into a sequence of numbers that each specify the amplitude of the speech signal at some instant of time. The procedure is analogous to producing the chart of Table 3.1 which recorded the variations of temperature. Digital computers, however, would record these numbers using a binary code in which number values on the base 10 that we commonly use are represented on the base 2. The number of "bits" in terms of which the input analog signal is "quantized" simply represents the number of "steps" or "gradations" available to the computer's analog-to-digital (A to D) converter which effects this process. A two-bit quantization would allow $2^2 = 4$ levels of amplitude to be coded. A five-bit quantization allows $2^5 = 32$ levels of amplitude to be coded. The more bits, the finer the gradations of amplitude that can be reproduced. Most speech analysis programs use ten- or eleven-bit quantization which allows the computer program to code 1024 or 2048 levels of amplitude. This degree of quantization is adequate for the analysis of speech. It would not suffice for music where 16 bits would be appropriate since the dynamic range, the difference between the quietest and loudest sounds that are of interest, is greater.

Sampling rate

The speech signal must be sampled at intervals of time. Table 3.1 presented measurements made at intervals of four hours. This slow sampling rate obviously would not suffice for the analysis of speech. Events that occur more rapidly must be sampled more frequently or else the event will come and go before it is observed. As we noted earlier, the concept of frequency captures the tempo of events. An acoustic signal that has energy at a frequency of 500 Hz contains energy that changes five times as fast as an acoustic signal that is limited to energy varying at a maximum frequency of 100 Hz. The Nyquest sampling theorem (Flanagan, 1972) states that a signal must be sampled at a rate that is at least twice the maximum frequency of interest in order to preserve significant temporal variations. In other words, if a speech signal contains information at 9 kHz that we believe is perceptually significant, we must sample at a rate of at least 18 000 samples per second. In practice we would sample at a rate of 20 000 samples per second to preserve information at 9 kHz. The process seems a bit circular, since we have to know the frequency range that is of interest before we can determine the sampling rate for speech analysis. However, science is cumulative and we can rely on past work. A sampling rate of 10 000 samples per second thus is appropriate for most acoustic analyses of the speech of adult humans. A rate of 20 000 samples per second is necessary for the analysis of children's speech which contains energy at higher frequencies. Signals like birdsong may require sampling rates of 32 000 to 40 000 samples per second.

You may ask, why not sample at the highest rate possible? The problem there is one of computer memory and computational time. The greater the sampling rate, the more space the sample takes up in the computer's electronic memory. Thus sampling at twice the rate takes up twice as much computer memory for the same sample duration. The algorithms that analyze the signal must also consider each stored sample sequentially. Hence they will take twice as much time to analyze a speech signal sampled at twice the rate of another. The sampling rate to be used in a given situation will thus depend on the frequency range of the signal that you wish to analyze, its duration, and the memory size and operating speed of the computer system being used.

Low-pass filtering
One additional precaution is necessary in the analog-to-digital process. The input signal *must* be low-pass filtered at the value of the highest frequency that you are analyzing–the frequency appropriate to your sampling rate. Thus, if you are sampling at 20 000 samples per second for the analysis of speech signals having energy at 9 kHz, you must use a low-pass filter at 9 kHz. If you neglect this step you will introduce "aliasing" artifacts (Rabiner and Schafer, 1979).

Setting the level
As we noted earlier in this chapter, it is necessary to avoid overloading and distorting the acoustic signal when you record it either as an analog signal in a conventional tape recorder or sound spectrograph, or as a digital signal. Figure 5.14A shows the waveform of the sound [ba] as it is displayed on the monitor scope of the BLISS system without distortion. Figure 5.14B shows a distorted recording of this waveform. The signal was played at a level that was too high into the computer's analog-to-digital converter. The peaks of the

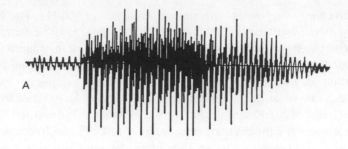

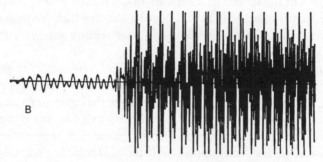

Figure 5.14. The waveform of the sound [ba] as it is displayed on the monitor of the BLISS system without distortion (top); the same waveform but recorded with distortion (bottom).

waveform were "clipped" off. A Fourier analysis of the clipped signal would show spurious high frequency energy. (Clipping introduces electrical energy that did not exist in the original signal.) The BLISS system and other speech analysis packages have "clipping" detectors that look for these distortion products. In the absence of distortion monitors, the digital version of the input signal should be visually monitored. You should also listen to the digital version of the input signal. It is often possible to hear the distortion products.

Analysis procedures

Waveform analysis

Digital computer systems enable accurate quantitative measurements of temporal events to be made. Figure 5.15 shows the waveform of a [ta] with two "cursors" placed on it. These cursors are manually positioned using a "light pen," a "mouse," or cursor controls on the keyboard controlling the computer program. The left cursor, L0, is positioned at the onset of the "burst" of energy

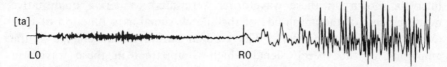

Figure 5.15. The waveform of a [ta] with cursor L0 representing the onset of the burst and R0 representing the start of phonation.

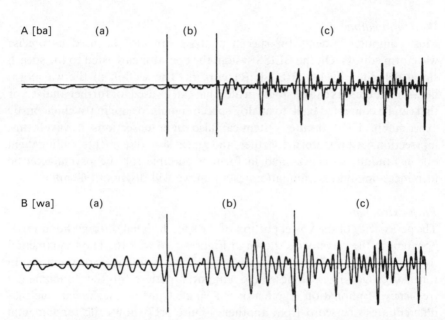

Figure 5.16. Waveforms for the sounds [ba] and [wa]. Letters indicate different acoustic segments demarcated by cursors: (a) prevoicing, (b) consonantal release, and (c) steady-steady portion of the vowel. (After Mack and Blumstein, 1983.)

that occurs when the speaker's tongue tip moves away from the teeth in the production of the sound [t]. The burst shows up as the sudden increase in the amplitude of the waveform. The right cursor, R0, is positioned at the start of phonation. The computer program has calculated the duration of the interval between cursors L0 and R0. This interval, the "voice onset time," is a significant cue in the perception of speech, differentiating sounds like [p], [t] and [k] from [b], [d], and [g]. The computer system facilitates the precise calculation of this linguistically significant measure.

Waveform measurements that reveal acoustic cues to linguistically signifi-cant events have yielded insights that would have otherwise been difficult to make. Figure 5.16 shows waveforms for the sounds [ba] and [wa]. The marked

81

intervals shown on these waveforms were used to derive quantitative measurements of the amplitude of the speech signal as a function of time (Mack and Blumstein, 1983). The gradual nature of the change in the amplitude of the speech signal which is apparent in these waveform measurements appears to be a significant acoustic cue to the linguistic distinction between the *stop consonant* [b] and the *glide* [w]. We will discuss this cue in more detail in Chapter 8.

Waveform editing

Most computer systems for speech analysis can also be used as precise waveform editors. On the BLISS system the operator can listen to the speech signal delimited by L0, R0, L1, R1 cursors. The section of the waveform between the cursors can be stored in files that can be used for further analysis or that can be converted back to analog speech signals for use in psychoacoustic experiments. The computer system can also reiterate sections of waveforms, join sections of a waveform together, and repeat stored segments, calling them out in random sequences and in formats suitable for the psychoacoustic identification and discrimination tests that we will discuss in Chapter 7.

Pitch extraction

The periodicity of the vowel portion of the speech signal during phonation is apparent in the waveforms shown in Figures 5.14 to 5.16. The fundamental frequency of phonation serves as an acoustic cue to linguistic distinctions. In tone languages like Chinese, the temporal pattern of the fundamental frequency of phonation or pitch over a single word is a *segmental* cue that differentiates one word from another. Figure 5.17 shows the fundamental frequency of phonation contours derived by the computer system for two words of Chinese spoken in isolation (Tseng, 1981). The computer system calculated the fundamental frequency of phonation between points in the waveform that the system operator had first marked with the cursors L0 and R0. The computer system in this case used an autocorrelation procedure (Flanagan, 1972) to calculate the fundamental frequency of phonation. The calculated fundamental frequency of phonation was displayed on the computer scope against the waveform; the system operator was able to intervene and readjust various parameters that are relevant to autocorrelation to avoid artifacts.

Pitch perturbations – jitter

Computer systems can be designed to follow rapid changes in the fundamental frequency of phonation. The display in Figure 5.18 shows a waveform in which the computer program has determined the duration of thirteen periods of the

82

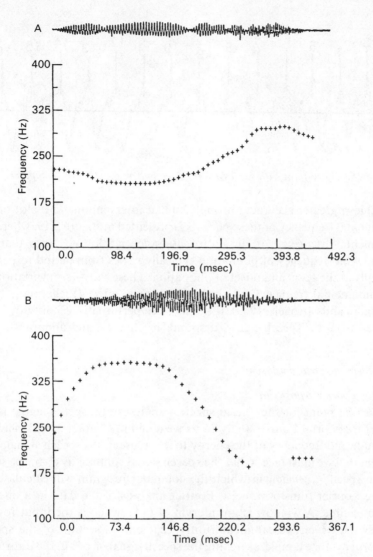

Figure 5.17. Waveforms and fundamental frequency of phonation for the vowel [i] in two words of Chinese spoken in isolation.

waveform during phonation. The indices are displayed for each period so that the operator can examine the waveform and enter corrections when the computer program does not correctly "mark" the period. The process of measuring the fundamental frequency of phonation typically introduces errors. Computer systems do not yet work as well as human beings for pattern recognition. By displaying the speech waveform and the calculated periods we

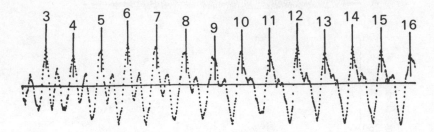

Figure 5.18. A waveform with successive pitch periods marked by the computer.

can achieve greater accuracy through human intervention. The plot of the fundamental frequency of these periods is presented in Figure 5.19, where the fundamental frequency of the entire utterance is plotted. Note that the fundamental frequency of phonation typically varies from period to period, especially at the onset and offset of phonation. These short-term variations in the fundamental frequency of phonation convey affect (Lieberman, 1961; Lieberman and Michaels, 1963). If these "pitch perturbations" or "jitter" are removed from the speech signal, it sounds mechanical and unnatural.

Short-term spectral analyses

Discrete Fourier transform

The starting point for short-term spectral analyses of a speech signal is the Fourier transform. Fourier analysis, as we noted in Chapter 3, will yield the amplitude and frequency of the energy that is present in a speech signal. One problem that we must face is that the speech signal continually changes, so we have to specify a *window* in which the computer program will calculate the discrete Fourier transform, i.e. a Fourier analysis of the data in a discrete sample of time. A window is an interval of time which is the input for the analysis. However, we cannot abruptly "cut out" a section of the speech waveform by, for example, switching the speech signal on or off. If we abruptly cut out a section of the waveform we would introduce high frequency noise that would in itself reflect the abrupt cut. Figure 5.20 shows a speech waveform for the vowel [i] on which we have positioned a window. The shape of this window is called a full-Hamming window. As you can see, it gradually tapers the energy that it allows to pass through as a function of time. The BLISS system can generate rectangular, Hamming, half-Hamming and Kaiser windows. The Hamming and Kaiser windows, which are both named after the people who mathematically explored their properties, are most often used for speech analysis. Technical details on these windows and the algorithms that

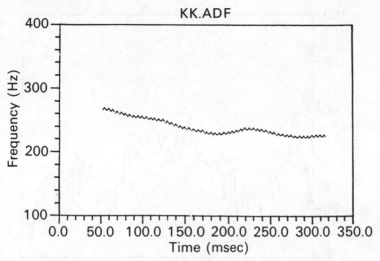

Figure 5.19. *A plot of the fundamental frequency of the word* dog *spoken by a three-month-old child. This includes the periods marked in Figure 5.18.*

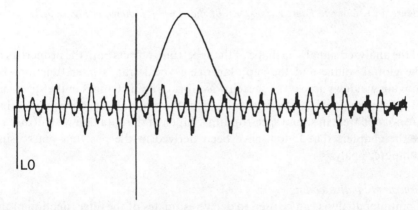

Figure 5.20. *A speech waveform for the vowel [i] with a full-Hamming window placed after the third pitch period.*

are relevant to speech analysis can be found in *Digital processing of speech* (Rabiner and Schafer, 1979).

Figure 5.21 shows the discrete Fourier transform that corresponds to the speech signal under the window shown in Figure 5.20. Note the small peaks that occur at approximately 110 Hz intervals. Nine peaks occur in a 1 kHz interval, i.e. every 110 Hz. (They actually occur every 111.1 Hz.) These peaks reflect the periodic nature of the rate at which the vocal cords of the larynx open and close – the fundamental frequency of phonation. The overall shape

85

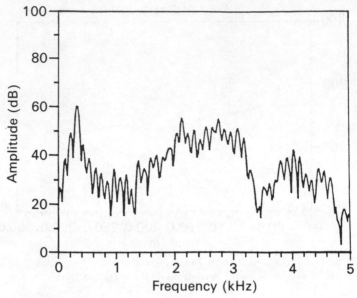

Figure 5.21. Discrete Fourier transform of the vowel [i] shown in Figure 5.20.

of the analyzed signal, the shape of the spectrum, reflects both the properties of the glottal source and the supralaryngeal vocal tract's filter function. By moving windows across the speech waveform, rapid changes in the spectrum of the speech signal can be detected (e.g. at the onset of stop consonants) that are not apparent in sound spectrograms. Much of the data that we will discuss in the chapters that follow have been derived in the past ten years using computer analysis.

Linear predictive coding

Computer analysis can be used to derive estimates of the filter function of the supralaryngeal vocal tract. Figure 5.22 shows an analysis of the same speech segment as Figure 5.21. The solid line that has been added to the display shows the estimated filter function derived by means of linear predictive coding (LPC) (Atal and Hanauer, 1971). The LPC algorithm takes account of some of the constraints of the acoustic theory of speech production that were noted by Fant (1960). The algorithm "knows" that human speech is produced by a supralaryngeal vocal tract that yields a number of formants or "poles" that have specified bandwidths. The computer program in effect matches the input spectrum against a library of formant frequency combinations. The algorithm selects the "best" match.

The computer operator using the **BLISS** system can specify the number of

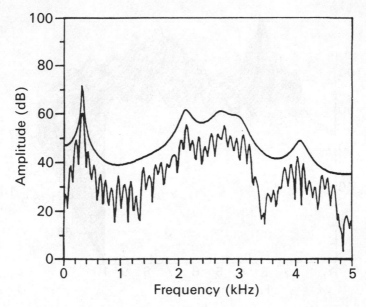

Figure 5.22. Formant frequencies have been derived for the speech sample under the window shown in Figure 5.20. The solid line was derived by an LPC program. The irregular line beneath it is a discrete Fourier transform which was plotted in Figure 5.21.

poles and bandwidths that the LPC algorithm will use to generate a matching signal. LPC analysis, like all human creations, can make errors. Most LPC algorithms assume an all-pole network. This can produce errors in the analysis of any speech sound that has zeros or antiformants in it, i.e. anything other than a nonnasalized vowel or [h]. Despite these limitations, LPC has been extremely useful in the analysis of the acoustic characteristics of speech and is commonly used by many researchers. The human operator can check the LPC analysis against the Fourier transform to avoid certain obvious errors, e.g. identifying the harmonics of a speech signal that has a high fundamental frequency of phonation as "formants." Note the peaks at 0.3, 2.1, 2.9, and 4.0 kHz which reflect the formant frequencies of the vowel [i] as produced by this speaker during the time interval defined by the window.

Displays like that of Figure 5.23 in which calculated filter functions are shown as a "three-dimensional" display are often useful since a formant frequency which shows as a "peak" in this display should not suddenly appear or vanish during the steady-state portion of a vowel. The three-dimensional display is also useful in that it shows the temporal pattern of formant frequency transitions as well as short-term onset cues. We will discuss these acoustic cues in the chapters that follow.

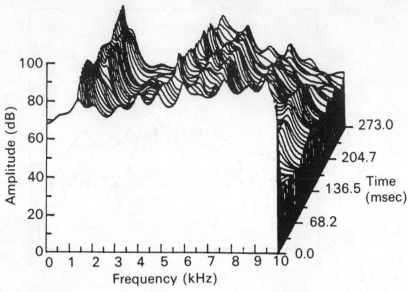

Figure 5.23. A three-dimensional display of the LPC spectrum for the vowel [i] shown in Figure 5.20.

The computer packages that have been developed for speech analysis also generally yield other analyses, e.g. plots of the energy of the acoustic signal as a function of time, plots of formant frequencies, spectral analysis in "critical" bands which analyze the acoustic waveform in terms of the properties of the auditory system, etc. The options vary for different packages and the user must follow the specific instructions for different packages. It is important to remember that whichever analysis package you are using, artifacts can occur that follow from interaction of the particular algorithms and the characteristics of the particular speech signal that is being analyzed. You must be suspicious and canny – the computer cannot think for you.

Exercises

We will conduct a speech analysis experiment that will illustrate some of the points that have been discussed in Chapter 5. The exercise can be completed if you have access to either a computer-implemented speech analysis system or a spectrograph, though certain aspects of speech are best analyzed using a computer.

1. Prepare a "script" for obtaining a tape recording for speech analysis. The script will be used by the subjects of the experiment. We will want each subject to produce three repetitions of the following English words:
    heed
    hid

who'd
peat
pat
bat
beet
boot
tea
gee

The following two sentences should also be on the list. They should also be repeated three times:

He's a good baby.
Is he really a baby?

You will have to make a list in which each test item appears followed by some other test item in a random-like manner. In other words, you do not want the speaker to simply repeat each item three times and then go on to the next item.

2. Make a tape recording of a male and a female speaker who have different fundamental frequencies of phonation reading your script. Follow the recommendations concerning recording level, noise, print-through, etc.

3. Derive the first two formant frequencies, F_1 and F_2, for the vowels of all the isolated words. Is it more difficult to derive the formant frequencies of the speaker who has a higher fundamental frequency f_0? Are the formant frequencies of the "same" vowel different for the two speakers?

4. Derive f_0 contours for the two sentences. What happens to f_0 at the end of each sentence? What sort of inter- and intra-speaker variation in f_0 do you find for the repetitions of the sentences?

6

Anatomy and physiology of speech production

In Chapter 5 we discussed the sound spectrograph in detail because it was for many years the primary instrument for speech analysis. Its limitations must be understood to see how theories for speech perception changed as computer-implemented analysis became possible. Our "knowledge" of the world ultimately depends on the quality of the data available, as do the theories that we formulate to interpret these data. Techniques like high-speed cinematography, radiographs (X-rays), cineradiographs, and electromyography have made new forms of data available which speech scientists and phoneticians have used to synthesize and test new theories. We will focus on these new techniques and data in this chapter as they bear on the anatomy and physiology of speech production. However, we also have to keep in touch with classical data and theories. The anatomical basis of speech production, for example, has been studied in much detail (Negus, 1949; Zemlin, 1968), and much of our understanding still rests on the classical techniques of anatomical observation and inference.

We will develop the systems approach that we introduced in Chapter 2. The subglottal, laryngeal, and supralaryngeal components of the vocal tract obviously must be treated as a complete system, but different experimental techniques are appropriate for the measurement of relevant physiological data on these components, and different physiological principles are necessary to understand how these systems function. The anatomical charts that we will present will bear a number of terms that identify various morphological features. Although these features must be labelled, our discussion will not necessarily involve all of these structures. It is necessary to know your way around the anatomy of the vocal tract because you cannot always predict what structures may become relevant as new studies investigate various aspects of speech production. However, it is not necessary to memorize all the names that appear on each chart. Hopefully you will begin to remember the important features as you follow the discussion.

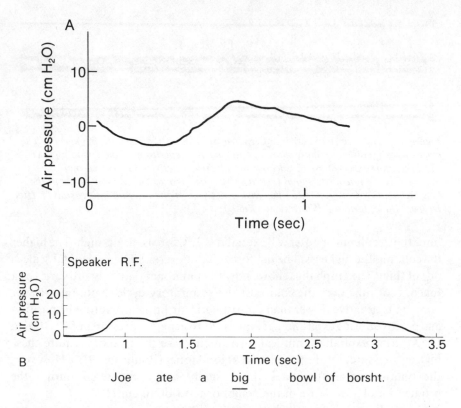

Figure 6.1. (A) Pulmonary air pressure during quiet respiration. (B) Pulmonary air pressure during speech. The speaker was instructed to emphasize the underlined word in the sentence. Note the air pressure peak.

The lungs

The discussion in Chapter 2 stressed the role of the elastic recoil force of the lungs. In normal inspiration the inspiratory muscles expand the lungs. Some of the force that is necessary for inspiration is stored in the elastic lungs. During expiration the elastic recoil of the lungs can provide the force necessary to push air out of the lungs. The bicycle pump and balloon model of Chapter 2 illustrated the dynamic behavior of the subglottal respiratory system, and we noted that maintaining a steady pulmonary air pressure during speech requires a complex pattern of muscular activity.

The two graphs in Figure 6.1 illustrate the resulting air pressure contours. Graph A shows pulmonary air pressure during "quiet" respiration, i.e. when the subject is not talking. The vertical scale is the air pressure in the lungs measured in centimetres of H_2O. Air pressure is often measured in terms of the

91

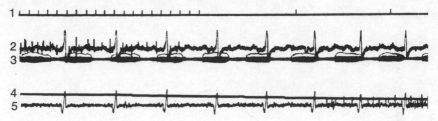

Figure 6.2. The electrical activity of several muscles of the chest during speech. The traces were recorded on an oscilloscope during the repetition of the syllable [ma]; (1) time marker, seconds; (2) decreasing electrical activity of the external intercostals; (3) acoustic signal recorded by microphone; (4) volume of air in the lungs gradually decreasing; (5) increasing activity of the internal intercostals. (After Draper, Ladefoged and Whitteridge, 1960.)

force that a column of water will exert if it is 2, 3, 5, 6.4 cm, etc. high. The higher the column, the higher will be the force that it exerts.[1] The horizontal scale is one of time. The graph thus shows how the pulmonary air pressure varies as a function of time over the course of the respiratory cycle. Note that the air pressure is negative (lower than atmospheric air pressure) during inspiration and positive during expiration. It is possible to generate pressures of 70–100 cm H_2O during expiration; musical instruments like the trumpet require these high air pressures for the production of loud tones (Bouhuys, 1974). However, the pulmonary air pressures that usually are encountered during the production of speech are in the neighborhood of 10 cm H_2O.

Graph B in Figure 6.1 shows the pulmonary air pressure during the production of speech. Note that the duration of the expiration in graph B has been extended to encompass a complete sentence. The speaker in this study was reading a long list of sentences. He typically produced each sentence on a complete expiration. Note that the overall shape of the air pressure functions plotted in the two graphs differs.

In Figure 6.2 a recording of the electrical activity of several of the muscles of the chest is reproduced (Draper, Ladefoged and Whitteridge, 1960). As we noted in Chapter 2, the regulation of air pressure during the production of speech involves a fairly complex sequence of muscular maneuvers. At the start of the expiration, the force of the elastic recoil of the lungs is very high. If the elastic recoil force were not opposed, the pulmonary air pressure would be much higher than 10 cm H_2O. The speaker whose muscle activity is monitored in Figure 6.2, therefore, initially opposed the elastic recoil force by tensing his external intercostal muscles. This shows up in line 2 of Figure 6.2 in terms of the height and number of electrical "spikes" recorded by the electrode that was

---

[1] Air pressures are traditionally measured in terms of the height a column of liquid, for example water or mercury, will exert.

inserted into this muscle. (The electrode was thinner than a standard hypodermic needle and is not itself dangerous or painful if inserted carefully. Medical supervision is, however, obviously mandatory for this procedure.)

The external intercostal muscle is an inspiratory muscle in the sense that it functions during quiet respiration to expand the lungs during inspiration. The speaker, however, is using this muscle during the expiratory phase of speech to "hold back" the elastic recoil force and maintain a steady low pulmonary air pressure. Note that the activity of this muscle, as indicated by the frequency and amplitude of the electrical spikes, diminishes, and that the speaker gradually brings into play an internal intercostal muscle. The internal intercostal muscle monitored is an expiratory muscle, i.e. it contracts to deflate the lungs and force air out of the respiratory system. The speaker brings this muscle into play to keep the pulmonary air pressure steady as the elastic recoil force falls below the level necessary to maintain the initial level. In other words, there is a complex patterning of muscles that is necessary to maintain a steady air pressure during speech. The "scheduling" of these different muscles will depend on the length of the sentence that the speaker intends to produce, and the speaker's posture. If you are standing erect, the contents of your stomach will pull downwards and tend to expand the lung volume. If you are flat on your back or in an intermediate position, a different pattern of muscular activity will be necessary to maintain the same pulmonary air pressure (Mead, Bouhays and Proctor, 1968). The demands imposed by the need for different oxygen transfer rates in walking or running also interact with the constraints of speech (Bouhuys, 1974), but speakers are able to make all the necessary adjustments "automatically."

Linguistic implications of respiratory control: syllable and sentence

Studies of the variation of pulmonary air pressure during speech (Draper, Ladefoged and Whitteridge, 1960; Lieberman, 1967, 1968; Atkinson, 1973) show that it is relatively steady over the course of a sentence-length expiration. There are no systematic variations that correspond to "syllable pulses" as Stetson (1951) claimed. Local "prominences" in air pressure sometimes occur when a speaker stresses or emphasizes a syllable or word, but this is not always the case (Lieberman, 1967, 1968; Atkinson, 1973). Different speakers, moreover, regulate their pulmonary air pressure in different manners. The single factor that is uniform is that the pulmonary air pressure must fall at the end of an expiration. This is obviously a necessary consequence of the speaker's initiating inspiration, which must involve a negative pulmonary air pressure. The terminal falling air pressure transitions in Figure 6.1 illustrate this phenomenon.

The control of the muscles of respiration is interesting because it demonstrates that the muscular gestures that underlie speech are "programmed," i.e. organized in a global manner in terms of linguistically determined segments. A speaker seems to have some knowledge of the duration of the sentence that he is going to utter before he takes air into his lungs. The amount of air that a speaker takes into his lungs is usually proportional to the length of the sentence that *will be* uttered. The duration of an expiration is thus linguistically conditioned during speech production and it can vary between 300 milliseconds and 40 seconds. It usually marks the length of a sentence. In the recitation of certain types of poetry it is a function of the poetic structure (Lieberman and Lieberman, 1973). This contrasts with the usual two-second length of the expiratory phase during quiet respiration. The inspiratory phase of respiration is roughly equal to the expiratory phase in duration during quiet breathing. During speech production or during the excitation of woodwind or brass instruments, the inspiratory phase stays short while the expiratory phase varies in duration. The physiology of the respiratory system that allows the inspiratory muscles to hold back the elastic recoil force of the lungs probably is the reason that speech takes place on the expiratory phase and the duration of the expiratory phase is the linguistically conditioned variable.

The physiology of the human subglottal respiratory system is not a uniquely human attribute. Its anatomy is essentially similar to that of other terrestrial mammals. The seemingly odd system in which the lungs essentially float in the pleural space (which gives rise to the elastic recoil force) follows from the fact that the lungs evolved from the swim bladders of fish (Darwin, 1859). Other animals, for example, wolves, whose vocal communications involve long passages of vocalization, also produce their calls on the expiratory phase of respiration.

Humans appear to use feedback control mechanisms to regulate their respiratory muscles during speech and singing. Feedback control systems are essentially ones in which the output of the system is monitored in order to make necessary corrections. In a feedback-regulated cookie factory, the final products would be constantly sampled and eaten. If their taste, texture, and so on, deviated from the desired standards of quality, necessary corrections would be taken at appropriate stages in the production process. In a feedback-regulated high fidelity amplifier for the reproduction of music, the electrical output of the amplifier is constantly monitored by means of electronic circuits that also apply signals that correct distortions. Feedback-regulated systems obviously differ with respect to how they are implemented, how they work, how fast they work, etc., but all feedback systems must have sensors that derive information on the output of the "device" that is to be regulated. The feedback

Intercostal muscle

Spinal cord

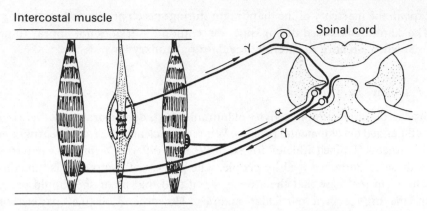

Figure 6.3. "Feedback" system for regulation of a respiratory muscle. (After Bouhuys, 1974.)

system also must transmit, or *feed*, this information *back* to some point where corrections can be made (hence the term *feedback*). In Figure 6.3 a schematic diagram of the intercostal muscles and a segment of the spinal cord illustrates some of the components of the feedback system that are involved in the regulation of respiration.

The middle muscle "fiber" in the diagram illustrates a *muscle spindle*. Muscle spindles are devices that signal the relative state of muscle contraction. A muscle applies a force as it contracts; its "output," therefore, is a function of the extent to which it has contracted. In Figure 6.3 the pathway labeled $\rightarrow\gamma$ transmits the electrical signal from the spindle to the spinal cord. At the level of the spinal cord special regulatory mechanisms generate electrical signals that are transmitted back to the intercostal muscles by the pathways labeled $\leftarrow\alpha$ and $\leftarrow\gamma$. The symbols α and γ identify particular pathways. The physiological function of these feedback systems in respiration is still not understood but it is clear that they play an essential role (Bouhuys, 1974). They operate extremely rapidly; the regulation of respiration as a function of exercise, for example, takes place within the phase of the breath in which work begins (Dejours, 1963).

Muscle spindles are numerous in the intercostal muscles, which, together with the abdominal muscles, are active during speech and singing. The diaphragm, which traditionally is supposed to be an important muscle for the regulation of pulmonary air pressure during singing, has very few muscle spindles. Despite the claims made by many teachers of voice and singing, the diaphragm performs no active role in either speech or singing (Bouhuys, 1974). The absence of muscle spindles and the role of feedback control perhaps

95

explain the inactivity of the diaphragm during speech production or singing. The diaphragm is used during quiet respiration but it does not appear to be used when we have to carefully regulate pulmonary air pressure.

"Learning" to breathe

Studies of the respiratory activity of human infants demonstrate that there is a well-defined developmental process. What is not clear is the role of learning in this process. Trained athletes, for example, have different respiratory patterns to those of untrained healthy people. The process of "learning" is "unconscious" in the sense that the athlete is not told that he or she should use a specific muscle in a particular manner. However, a distinct pattern of "learned" activity emerges as the athlete is exposed to a particular environmental situation. The process by which we learn to produce the sounds of a particular language or dialect is not conceptually different from the process by which an athlete learns to breathe while running. We do not know what we are doing when we learn to talk. We simply learn to speak a language if we are exposed to the linguistic environment and start before we are too old. There appears to be a critical period or critical periods involved in language learning. If we start before a certain age (which may vary for different individuals), it is easy to learn to speak a second language fluently. For most people it becomes impossible or extremely difficult to learn to speak another language without a "foreign accent" after a certain age. Similar effects occur with respect to the "simple" act of breathing. Human beings appear to "learn" how to breathe effectively at high altitudes. If you are a native "lowlander" who ascends to 12 500 feet, exercise is at first very difficult. If you wait and acclimatize, after approximately 11 days, your respiratory pattern changes and it becomes easier to exercise. However, the native "highlanders," who have grown up living at that altitude, breathe more effectively (LeFrancois *et al.*, 1969). They need to take in about 50 percent less air than you do when you and they perform the same task. The ability to learn the respiratory patterns that lead to more effective breathing at high altitudes appears to involve a critical period. Many of the coordinated patterns of muscular activity that structure various aspects of the behavior of humans and other animals appear to involve learning an automatic response pattern (Bouhuys, 1974; Lieberman, 1975).

The measurement of lung volume and volume change

We have already discussed some of the techniques that are necessary to derive data on pulmonary air pressure during speech or singing. Measurements of lung volume and the rate of change of lung volume which is equivalent to air flow are easy to get without much discomfort to the subject. As the volume of air in your lungs increases or decreases, the volume of your body also increases or decreases. There is no "excess space" within your body. You can therefore measure changes in lung volume by measuring changes in the volume of your body that occur as you breathe. You could, in theory, do this by using the same procedure that Archimedes used several thousand years ago. If you immersed your body in a bathtub and breathed with only your head and one hand out of the water you would notice that the level of the water rose slightly when you inflated your lungs. You could mark the water level on the bathtub with a marker and see the fall in level as you produced a long sentence, perhaps shouting "Eureka!" at its end. The volume of your body increases as you take air in and you will therefore displace more water at the start of a sentence than at its end.

The device that is usually used to measure lung volume is called the *body plethysmograph*. It consists of a sealed box in which a subject can sit with his head out and a seal around his neck. The air inside the box will be disturbed as the volume of the subject's body changes as he breathes in and out. It is not difficult to measure these changes in the air trapped inside the plethysmograph and compute the changes in lung volume (Bouhuys, Proctor and Mead, 1966). It is not necessary to put a face mask on the subject or otherwise to interfere with his breathing.

The body box or plethysmograph, however, will not respond to rapid changes in air flow. The rapid changes in air flow that are associated with sounds like the consonants [p], [t], or [h] can be measured with face masks that incorporate wire mesh flowmeter screens (Klatt, Stevens and Mead, 1968). Other procedures can be used to measure lung volume and air flow by relating the expansion of the rib cage and abdomen to the volume of the lungs (Hixon, Goldman and Mead, 1973).

The larynx

The larynx is an air valve that has two basic modes of operation. It can be set to a particular sized opening, which can vary from a complete closure of the airway from the lungs to minimum obstruction. The larynx is generally open widest during inspiration, when it is advantageous to have minimum interference with the air flow. The pictures of the larynx in Chapter 2 showed the larynx in an open position. The larynx can completely seal the airways. This frequently occurs when you are standing erect and lifting a weight. The larynx closes and seals air in the lungs, which stabilizes the rib cage. The larynx can also close to protect the lungs from the intrusion of harmful material. The larynx maintains particular openings during the production of certain speech

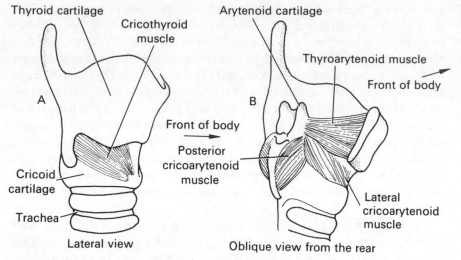

Figure 6.4. Cartilages and intrinsic muscles of the larynx.

sounds. We will discuss data that show that the larynx opens wider during the production of a sound like [h] than it does during a sound like [f] (the first sound of the word *fat*). However, the speech function that the larynx is most directly associated with is the generation of quasi-periodic series of puffs of air. These periodic, or nearly periodic, air puffs constitute the source of acoustic energy that characterizes phonation. As we noted in Chapter 2, the vowels of English are usually phonated or, in the terminology that is usually used in linguistically oriented discussions, *voiced*.

The myoelastic-aerodynamic theory of phonation

In Figure 6.4 several views are sketched of the cartilages and intrinsic muscles of the human larynx. It is very difficult to visualize the larynx's separate parts. Our knowledge of how the larynx works derives from Johannes Müller's nineteenth-century studies. Müller excised larynges from human cadavers, simulated the forces of various muscles by applying forces through strings fixed to various cartilages, and provided power to the system by blowing through the excised larynges (Müller, 1848). Van den Berg (1958, 1960, 1962) has quantitatively replicated Müller's original experiments.

The major structures of the larynx consist of a number of cartilages. Let us start from the bottom part of the larynx and work upwards. The first major cartilage is the *cricoid*, which is ring-shaped and sits on top of the trachea (Figure 6.4A). The trachea looks like a vacuum cleaner hose in most

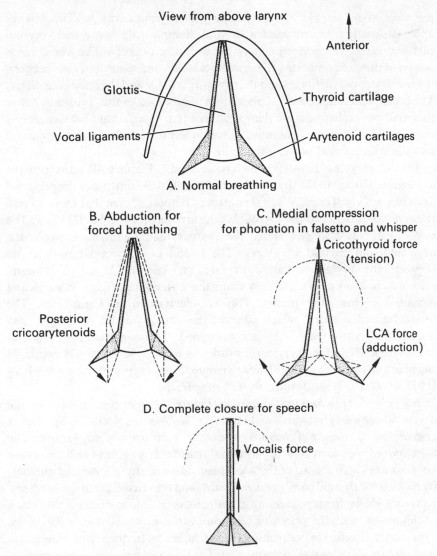

Figure 6.5. Action of the intrinsic laryngeal muscles (the term vocalis *is often applied to the thyroarytenoid muscle). (After Atkinson, 1973.)*

illustrations. Two small cartilages, the *arytenoids*, each sit on one side of the cricoid towards its posterior (rear) (Figure 6.4B). The relationship between the arytenoid cartilages and the muscles that operate on them may be somewhat clearer in the schematic views that appear in Figure 6.5. The *thyroid* cartilage also sits on top of the cricoid. It is open at the rear and its closed solid front surface is positioned on the anterior (front) surface of the cricoid. When you feel your Adam's apple you are feeling your thyroid cartilage. The Adam's apple is usually more prominent in adult human males since their thyroid cartilages grow disproportionately large during puberty. The vocal cords consist of the conglomerate of ligaments, muscles, and tissue that runs between the two arytenoid cartilages and the thyroid cartilage and the cricoid cartilage. The fundamental frequency of phonation of adult males thus is usually lower than that of females because their vocal cords are longer and heavier. As we shall see, heavier vocal cords move slower in response to the aerodynamic and aerostatic forces that power phonation.

The thyroarytenoid muscle, which is sketched in Figure 6.4B, runs from the arytenoid cartilage to the thyroid. It is the muscle that constitutes the principal mass of each vocal cord. When it contracts, it applies force that tends to pull the arytenoids closer to the thyroid, as the arrows on Figure 6.5D show. The vocal ligaments also run above the thyroarytenoid muscles between the arytenoid and thyroid cartilages. The lateral cricoarytenoid muscles go between the arytenoid cartilages and the cricoid. When the lateral cricoarytenoid muscles tense, they swing the arytenoid cartilages inwards and *adduct*, i.e. close, the glottis. This is schematized in Figure 6.5. The interarytenoid muscles, which connect the two arytenoid cartilages, also adduct the glottis when they are tensioned. The combination of lateral cricoarytenoids and interarytenoids function to pull the arytenoid cartilages together and close the glottis. These two muscles also apply what Van den Berg (1958, 1960, 1962) has termed *medial compression*.

The posterior cricoarytenoid muscle (Figure 6.4B), in contrast, swings the arytenoid cartilages outwards and opens, i.e. *abducts*, the glottis. The posterior cricoarytenoid muscle functions whenever you open your larynx. The cricothyroid muscle applies longitudinal tension. It lengthens and tenses the vocal cords (which consist of the vocal ligaments and thyroarytenoid muscles) by rocking the thyroid cartilage downwards and the cricoid cartilage upwards. Johannes Müller in his pioneering experiments was able to simulate the action of this muscle with the primitive technology that was available in the 1820s. This muscle is active in controlling the fundamental frequency of phonation, but is not its sole muscular determinant. The thyroarytenoids (vocalis muscle) upon contraction can either decrease or increase the tension in the vocal ligaments themselves, depending on the state of other muscles.

The forces of phonation

During phonation, the vocal cords move in response to a rapid alternation of aerodynamic and aerostatic forces generated by the flow of air. These forces are inherently nonlinear; they rapidly build up and then abruptly stop. The elastic forces of the larynx also interact with these forces during phonation.

The basis of phonation is, however, the passive movement of the vocal cords under the influence of forces generated by the movement of air outwards from the lungs. The larynx itself adds no energy to the process. The laryngeal muscles serve to initiate and modulate phonation. The dynamic interaction of the aerodynamic, aerostatic, and muscle forces during phonation is very complex and is the focus of research projects that make use of computer-modeling techniques (Flanagan *et al.*, 1970; Flanagan, Ishizaka and Shipley, 1975; Rothenberg, 1981). However, it is useful to discuss qualitatively the process of phonation in order to get a sense of the process. Phonation is initiated by the laryngeal muscles swinging the arytenoid cartilages together and setting an initial phonation neutral position, medial compression, and longitudinal tension for the vocal cords. The interarytenoid and lateral cricoarytenoid muscles adduct, i.e. bring the vocal cords together and keep them medially compressed. Medial compression is necessary in some degree for phonation to take place. Imagine bringing your lips together and squeezing them together slightly. You have adducted your lips and applied some medial compression. If you now blow air out from your lungs, you can start your lips moving rapidly outwards and then inwards, producing a raspy noise, if you have applied the right amount of medial compression.

If you squeeze your lips together too hard, they will stay closed. This is analogous to the production of a *glottal stop*, in which a great deal of medial compression is applied, stopping phonation. If, in contrast, you do not apply enough medial compression then you will simply blow your lips apart as you build up pulmonary air pressure. This is analogous to the production of turbulent or *strident* phonation. Newborn infants frequently do this, producing a characteristic quality to their cries. Strident phonation does not appear to be a phonetic feature of English, but it could be used. One point to remember here is that cutting back on medial compression is only one possible way of generating strident phonation. We will point out some other articulatory possibilities.

Now suppose that your vocal cords have swung together, partially or completely obstructing the air flow through the vocal tract. What happens? In Figure 6.6 a schematic view of a section made on a frontal plane is presented. A larynx in this plane is one sectioned from ear hole to ear hole with the saw blade running between the ear holes and then cutting down through the neck.

The arrows labeled F_{as} represent the aerostatic force generated by the air pressure impinging on the lower surface of the vocal cords. It is greatest when the cords are most nearly closed since $F_{as} = P_{pulmonary} \times A$ where $P_{pulmonary}$ is the pulmonary pressure and A is the surface area of the vocal cords. The arrow labeled F_b represents the negative air pressure generated by the Bernoulli force. This negative air pressure will pull the vocal cords together. The Bernoulli force is a consequence of the increase in the speed of the air molecules as they

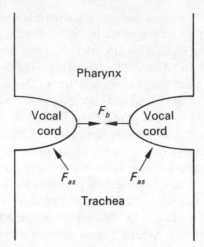

Figure 6.6. Schematic view of vocal cords and some of the forces of phonation.

move through the glottal constriction. As the glottal opening becomes smaller, the speed of the air molecules increases relative to their speed in the trachea and pharynx. The effect is similar to the motion of people when a crowd goes through a revolving door. When you are in the revolving door you are moving faster than you were in the crowd next to the door. The Bernoulli force is greatest when the glottal opening is smallest, except that it disappears, i.e. equals zero, when the glottis closes completely because there then is no air flow whatsoever (Lieberman, 1967). Phonation is the result of the process wherein vocal cords are moved in and out by these alternating forces that ultimately depend on the air pressure generated in the lungs, the pulmonary air pressure. F_{as} pushes the vocal cords apart. F_b sucks them together.

The laryngeal muscles position the vocal cords and provide the medial compression that keeps the vocal cords from being blown apart or simply staying sealed. The laryngeal muscles also set up a "tissue" force that enters into the balance of forces that produce phonation. The tissue force will always act to restore the vocal cord to its phonation neutral position. It is analogous to the force exerted by the spring on a screen door. The screen door's spring acts to pull the door back to its "neutral" position when it is opened. If a simplified equation of motion is derived for the vocal cords, the important relationship that governs the rate at which the vocal cords move in and out becomes apparent.

$$F_{as} - F_b - F_t = ma$$

where m is the mass of the vocal cords, a is the acceleration, and F_t is the tissue force.

102

At the start of a glottal cycle the glottal opening is small because the phonation neutral position has closed or nearly closed the glottis. F_{as} is maximum. If F_{as} is greater than the sum of F_t and F_b, the vocal cords move outwards. The glottal opening becomes larger and F_b decreases, but F_{as} also decreases and F_t increases. When F_t is greater than F_{as}, the vocal cords begin to move inwards, and the process repeats itself.

What will increase the acceleration a of the vocal cords? Obviously the acceleration will vary as the various forces change their magnitude during the glottal cycle. However, if the individual forces are greater, the acceleration will be greater in some part of the cycle. Thus, increasing the tissue force or increasing the pulmonary air pressure will increase the acceleration. (F_{as} is a function of the pulmonary air pressure.) The tissue force can be increased by tensing muscles like the lateral cricoarytenoid and interarytenoids, which generate medial compression, or by tensing the cricothyroid muscle, which stretches the vocal cords in their anterior–posterior plane (longitudinal tension). The thyroarytenoid muscles, which constitute the body of the vocal cords, will also increase the tissue force as they tense. So will the external thyroarytenoid muscles. Any one of a number of muscles can increase the tension on the vocal cords. So long as the vocal cords are phonating – this is important since the entire process can be stopped if some tension is set wrong, blowing the vocal cords apart or keeping them together — increases in tissue force will cause an increase in the acceleration of the vocal cords.

Since the velocity of the vocal cords is equal to the integral of acceleration with respect to time, the vocal cords will move faster if any of these forces increase. The fundamental frequency of phonation, which is the rate at which the vocal cords open and close, will thus increase if either the pulmonary air pressure or the tension set by the various laryngeal muscles increases. The laryngeal muscles as they tense can also change the vibrating mass that moves (Hollien and Curtis, 1960; Hollien, 1962; Hollien and Colton, 1969). If the forces that act on the vocal cords stay constant while the vibrating mass increases, the vocal cords will move more slowly. The lower average fundamental frequencies of phonation of adult males follow from the increased mass of their longer vocal cords (Peterson and Barney, 1952; Hollien, 1962). In sum, the fundamental frequency of phonation is a function of both the air pressure and the tension set by various laryngeal muscles.

Control of fundamental frequency: electromyographic data

Electromyographic data can be derived from the larynges of normal speakers by carefully inserting electrodes in appropriate muscles and amplifying and recording the signals (Sawashima, 1974). Electromyography is the study of the electrical activity of the muscles. The techniques for inserting the electrodes are very complex and must be approached with the greatest caution by otolaryngologists trained in this technique. In Figure 6.7 electromyographic data for the cricothyroid muscle and the sternohyoid muscle (one of the laryngeal "hanger" muscles which we will discuss in the next section of this chapter) are presented together with a record of the subglottal air pressure obtained by means of a tracheal puncture, and the audio signal. The speaker was an adult speaker of American English who was reading (with stress on the word *Bev*) the sentence *Bev loves Bob*. The fundamental frequency of phonation can be clearly seen both in the trace of subglottal air pressure and in the audio signal. Note that there is an increase in the subglottal air pressure on the initial stressed word *Bev*. If the speaker had not stressed this word, the subglottal air pressure would have been about 8 to 10 cm H_2O. There was also increased electrical activity in the cricothyroid muscle, which correlated with the stressed word. The electrical activity of the cricothyroid muscle shows up in terms of the amplitude and frequency of the "spikes." Note that the subglottal air pressure falls at the end of this expiration while phonation is still taking place. The fundamental frequency of phonation also falls as the subglottal air pressure falls.

The "raw" electromyographic data of Figure 6.7 are difficult to interpret. It is hard to make quantitative statements concerning the relative activity of particular muscles or the total pattern of muscular activity. The electrical activity that the electromyographic electrodes record can also be misleading if only one token of an utterance is considered. Various artifacts can be recorded and the speaker may also produce a particular token in an anomalous manner. The most reliable technique for the evaluation of electromyographic data makes use of computer-implemented averaging of a large sample of tokens of a particular utterance from an individual speaker. The speaker reads a long list of utterances that includes many tokens of particular sentences. The particular sentences are read in a random order to avoid the "singsong" patterns that can occur when you repeat an identical sentence over and over again. The electromyographic signals and the acoustic signal are continuously monitored and recorded on magnetic tape using a multitrack instrumentation recorder. Special marker signals are also recorded that identify the individual tokens of each sentence in the computer program that is later used to integrate the electromyographic signals derived from the muscles under investigation and average the integrated data for the many tokens of each particular sentence. The integrating and averaging process reduces the possibility of electrical artifacts being interpreted as muscle activity (Harris, 1974).

In Figure 6.8 computer-averaged data for 38 tokens of the sentence *Bev loves Bob* are presented. The same speaker produced all of these utterances in two

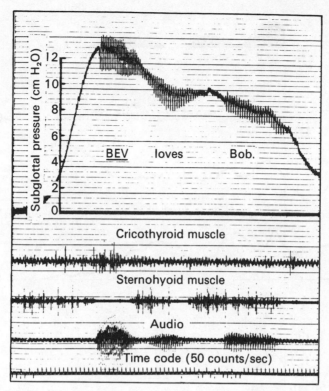

Figure 6.7. Subglottal air pressure, acoustic signal, and electromyographic activity of cricothyroid and sternohyoid muscles. (After Atkinson, 1973.)

different recording sessions. The plot of fundamental frequency as a function of time that appears at the bottom of Figure 6.8 was derived by a special computer program (Atkinson, 1973, p.38) that uses an autocorrelation method and is accurate to within 2 Hz. The integrated and averaged plots for three muscles are shown in this figure, which is derived from Atkinson (1973). Atkinson also measured the electrical activity of the sternohyoid and sternothyroid as well as subglottal air pressure, lung volume, and air flow. Note that there is a peak in the cricothyroid muscle's activity, which is correlated with the peak in fundamental frequency for the stressed word *Bev*. The lower fundamental frequency of the rest of the sentence, i.e. the words *loves Bob*, is a consequence of lower activity of the lateral cricoarytenoid muscle acting in concert with the cricothyroid and the subglottal air pressure (which was plotted in Figure 6.7).

Figure 6.9 shows plots of these muscles and fundamental frequency for the same speaker reading the question *Bev loves Bob?*. Note that the fundamental

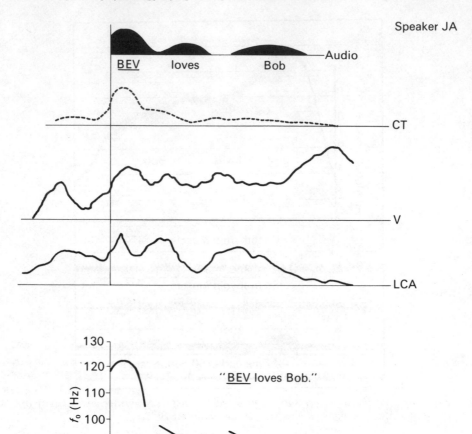

Figure 6.8. Computer-averaged and computer-integrated electromyographic signals and fundamental frequency of phonation as functions of time for 38 tokens of the sentence Bev loves Bob *spoken by one speaker. The speaker stressed the word* Bev. *The activity of the cricothyroid muscles (CT), internal thyroarytenoid muscles (V), and lateral cricoarytenoid muscles (LCA) electrical activity are plotted. (After Atkinson, 1973.)*

frequency rises sharply at the end of the sentence, when all three of the muscles show increased activity. A detailed statistical analysis by Atkinson correlating electromyographic data, subglottal air pressure, and f_0 changes shows that in utterances like that plotted in Figure 6.8 the fundamental frequency of phonation is primarily controlled by the subglottal air pressure. Although

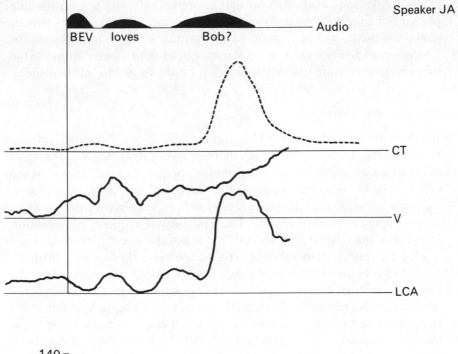

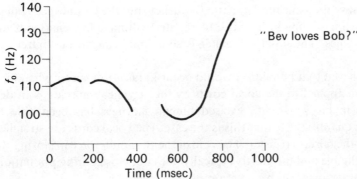

Figure 6.9. Plots similar to those of Figure 6.8 for the same speaker's tokens of the question Bev loves Bob?.

laryngeal muscles can be used to enhance the local prominences in the fundamental frequency function that are associated with the speaker's stressing a particular word (the word *Bev* in Figure 6.8), the primary determinant of f_0 variation is the subglottal air pressure. These utterances are produced with the larynx adjusted in a *register of phonation* that results in the fundamental frequency being fairly sensitive to air pressure variations. In contrast, Atkinson's analysis shows that in utterances like the yes–no question plotted in Figure 6.9 the larynx was not very sensitive to variations in sub-glottal air pressure. The fundamental frequency contour throughout this sentence is primarily a function of the tension of the laryngeal muscles; the subglottal air pressure has very little effect on the fundamental frequency.

Registers of phonation

Johannes Müller in the course of his pioneering studies with excised larynges found that the registers of phonation that singers had discerned were the result of the larynx phonating in different "modes." Singers had noted the presence of at least two basic modes of phonation, the "chest" and "falsetto" registers. A person singing in the falsetto register sounds quite different from the same person singing in the chest register. The fundamental frequency of phonation is higher in the falsetto register, but that is not the sole difference in voice quality. There is less energy present in the harmonics of the fundamental in the falsetto register than is the case of the chest register. A singer phonating at the same fundamental frequency in his falsetto register will have less energy present at higher harmonics of the fundamental than a singer phonating at the same fundamental in his or her chest register. A countertenor singing at the same fundamental as a contralto thus will have a different voice quality. Both singers will have the same fundamental frequency, but the glottal spectrum of the countertenor singing in his falsetto register will have less energy at the higher harmonics. The falsetto register is sometimes said to be "purer" in quality.

Müller believed that phonation would occur in falsetto register when high tensions were applied to the vocal cords by the laryngeal muscles. Van den Berg (1960) in his work with excised human larynges has been able to demonstrate quantitatively that this is the case. The vocal cords are stretched quite thin in the falsetto register. The role of the Bernoulli force in closing the glottis is negligible and the glottis typically does not close during phonation. The glottal waveform can become almost sinusoidal.

The "chest" register, which really does not involve using the chest in any unique way, may consist of several subregisters. The larynx does not behave in the same manner throughout the chest register. Van den Berg (1960) first noted that the sensitivity of the larynx to variations in subglottal air pressure varied for different adjustments of the laryngeal muscles. In other words, a change of, for example, 1 cm H_2O subglottal air pressure could result in a change as little as 2.5 Hz or as much as 18 Hz in the fundamental frequency, depending on how the vocal cords were positioned and tensioned. Van den Berg's data were derived from excised human larynges, so there was some question whether the muscular adjustments of this data actually occur in living human speakers.

Measurements on the rate of change in fundamental frequency with respect to changes in subglottal (or transglottal) air pressure in living speakers are, however, consistent with Van den Berg's data (Lieberman *et al.*, 1969; Ohala, 1970; Shipp, Doherty and Morrisey, 1979).

The muscular maneuvers that are involved in adjusting the larynx to achieve phonation in different registers are not completely understood. It looks as though the muscles that support the larynx are involved as well as the "intrinsic" muscles like the cricothyroid, interarytenoids, etc. These muscles help to support the cartilages of the larynx. They can also move the larynx with respect to other parts of the body. The sternohyoid muscle (cf. Figure 6.14), for example, can pull the larynx downward if the muscles that connect the hyoid bone to the mandible and skull are not tensioned. A number of studies have measured the activity of the sternohyoid muscle and have attempted to correlate its activity with the fundamental frequency of phonation. Some have found that fundamental frequency tended to fall when it was active (Ohala, 1970; Ohala and Hirose, 1970), whereas others have not (Garding, Fujimura and Hirose, 1970; Simada and Hirose, 1970). Atkinson's statistical analysis (1973) of the activity of the laryngeal muscles may explain these different results. The sternohyoid appears to function as a phonation register-shifting mechanism in the speakers whom he studied. The utterance plotted in Figure 6.8 was produced in what Atkinson terms the *low chest* register. The utterance plotted in Figure 6.9 was produced in the *high chest* register. The speaker appears to adjust his larynx to "set it up" in the appropriate register before he produces a sound. The sternohyoid muscle was active in Atkinson's data when the larynx was going through these register shifts. Studies in which the height of the larynx was compared to the fundamental frequency of phonation also demonstrate that lowering the larynx does not necessarily lower the fundamental frequency (Maeda, 1976).

The fry register
Much more research is necessary before we can state with reasonable certainty the muscular adjustments that are involved in effecting register shifts (Shipp and McGlone, 1971). Different individuals may use very different maneuvers, and some register shifts may be more natural or prevalent than others. Trained singers, for example, are able to make smooth transitions from one register to another by means of adjustments that may involve bending their necks and upper torsos (Proctor, 1964). The old photos of Caruso often show him with his chin pulled sharply downwards. Some registers of phonation are not commonly used by speakers of English. The *fry* register appears to involve very slack tension and a large vibrating mass. Ingenious radiographic techniques reveal the vibrating mass (Hollien and Colton, 1969). The fundamental frequency of phonation in this register is in the order of 60 Hz for a male

speaker but it can probably go lower. Children under age three years typically use the fry register during normal speech production and can phonate as low as 30 Hz (Keating and Buhr, 1978). Though children in this age range have much higher average fundamental frequencies, between 250 and 540 Hz, the range of variation of fundamental frequency is much greater than that of adults (Robb and Saxman, 1985). The fry register also shows a great deal of irregularity from one pitch period to the next. In certain pathological conditions associated with cancer of the larynx the fry register is all that a speaker can use (Lieberman, 1963; Hecker and Kreul, 1971).

Breathy phonation
During normal phonation the glottal waveform has energy only at the fundamental frequency and its harmonics. Noiselike "breathy" excitation of the vocal tract can, however, be generated by increasing the air flow through the larynx to the point where turbulence is generated. This can be done by introducing an opening that stays open throughout the glottal cycle (Timcke, Von Leden and Moore, 1958). If you think best in hydraulic terms, think of the larynx during phonation as a water valve that is being rapidly opened and closed, producing "puffs" of water. Opening a second valve and letting it stay open will increase the total air flow. There are several ways to do this. During normal phonation the larynx's posterior portion is held together while phonation takes place in the anterior portion. Looking down at the larynx, one sees the situation that is pictured in Figure 6.10A. If the posterior part is kept open during phonation as pictured in Figure 6.10B, a constant "shunt" will admit air through it. It is possible to open the posterior part by not tensioning the interarytenoid muscles. The glottal area waveform will be like that shown in Figure 6.11. Note that there is a constant steady opening through the larynx in addition to the periodic component.

The effect of the different phonation neutral positions of Figures 6.10B and 6.10C will be equivalent in so far as both maneuvers will yield additional air flow. The high air flow will generate turbulent noise excitation if the air flow in any part of the supralaryngeal vocal tract or at the larynx exceeds a critical air velocity. The effect is therefore abrupt or "quantal" (Stevens, 1972b). Turbulence is either present or not present.

In a sound like [h] the air flow at the glottis is itself so great that noise-like excitation is generated. "Normal" English vowels may also be produced using breathy excitation generated at the larynx. Whispered vowels *without* phonation have this quality. It is also possible to produce sounds in which both breathy and periodic excitation co-occur. This is often the case for whispered speech in normal subjects. It also may be the case for breathy vowels that occur in other languages.

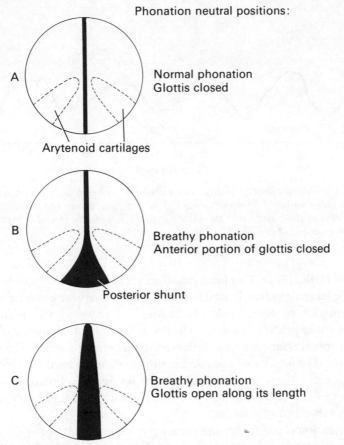

Figure 6.10. Adjustments of the larynx that can produce normal (A) and breathy phonation (B and C).

The production of voiceless sounds

Studies of the total air flow through the vocal tract show that voiced sounds are produced with significantly less air flow than voiceless sounds. Sounds like [h] and [s] are produced with the greatest air flow; voiceless stops like [p] with slightly less air flow. All of these voiceless sounds are, however, produced with significantly greater air flow than the voiced vowels (Klatt, Stevens and Mead, 1968). The terms − *voiced* and *voiceless* can be used interchangeably to denote sounds that are produced with noise sources without any periodic phonation occurring. The distinction inherent in the quantal contrast + *voicing* versus − *voicing* (or *voiced* versus *voiceless*) is binary. We are saying that sounds can be either voiced or unvoiced and that there is no intermediate state (Jakobson,

111

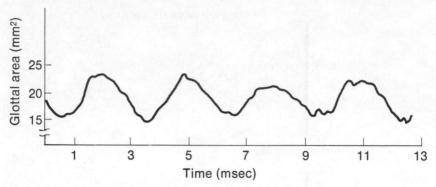

Figure 6.11. Measurement of glottal area waveform derived from computer analysis of a high-speed movie (Lieberman, 1963). The waveform shows the glottal opening as a function of time. Note that the glottis is never completely closed in this particular example of breathy phonation.

Fant and Halle, 1963). This binary distinction has a physiological basis in so far as the larynx can be adjusted either to yield phonation when air begins to flow through it or not to yield phonation. The physiological or functional contrast is thus inherently binary. However, the individual muscular maneuvers that are necessary to adjust the larynx so that phonation will take place are not binary. The activity of a particular muscle depends on the activity of the total ensemble of muscles that adjusts the larynx for phonation. It is not possible to derive a simple, binary muscle gesture that can be directly and uniquely related to phonation.

The situation is similar for the seemingly "simple" state of − *voicing*. The differences in air flow that are typical of the different sounds of speech are the result of subtle, graded adjustments of the glottal opening. Observations of the glottis derived from flexible fiber-optic bundles (which allow the larynx to be photographed during the production of normal speech)[2] show that the larynx opens more for the production of an [s] than for a [p] (Sawashima and

[2] The fiber-optic bundle consists of a set of thin fiberglass filaments. Each filament conducts a beam of light along its length in the same manner as a plastic wand conducts light around corners. The fiber-optic has thousands of filaments that each lie in a parallel, geometrically fixed relationship to the others. A lens projects an image on one end of the bundle and the image is conducted to the other end around bends, etc., to a camera (Sawashima and Hirose, 1968). The bundles are quite thin and flexible. If the bundles are inserted through the speaker's nose it will not interfere with articulatory maneuvers in the mouth. Other techniques for deriving information on the size of the glottis involve measuring the light that passes through. (A source of light is placed in contact with the speaker's throat against the front of the trachea and a photocell that picks up light is lowered to a position above the larynx (Ohala, 1966; Lisker, Cooper and Schvey, 1969)). This method, however, can introduce many artifacts. Ultrasonic scanning techniques (Minifie, Kelsey and Hixon, 1968) and methods that measure the electrical resistance of the glottis have also been used with varying degrees of success (Sawashima, 1974).

Miyazaki, 1973). Electromyographic data furthermore show that the different-sized glottal opening is the result of a deliberate muscular maneuver (Hirose and Ushijama, 1974). It is not a secondary result of the greater air flow of the sound [s]. The speaker, in other words, deliberately opens his glottis a little wider to produce greater air flow for the sound [s]. The greater air flow is necessary to generate noise at the constriction that is formed near the speaker's teeth in the production of the sound [s]. The size of this constriction is greater for an [s] than it is for a [p] for the interval in which noise must be generated. It takes more air to generate noise at a constriction through air turbulence when the constriction is wider (Flanagan, 1972). Noise will be generated at a constriction only if the air flow in the constriction is in excess of a critical value. If the constriction is small, the average air flow through the vocal tract does not need to be as high as when the constriction is relatively large. That is because the air flow is more concentrated in the constricted portion if the constriction is smaller.[3]

The "binary" quality of voicing as a phonetic contrast thus rests in the acoustic consequences of the total speech producing mechanism. In producing a "simple" − *voiced* sound the speaker takes into account the relative size of the constriction of the upper airway at which the noise excitation will be generated. At the articulatory and muscular levels (the levels that correspond to data derived by observing structures like the larynx or by monitoring the electrical activity of particular muscles), speech production is complex and no element of the vocal tract operates in an independent manner.

Our discussion of the binary nature of the sound contrast *voicing* would not be complete if we did not note that some sounds, e.g. the sound [z] in the word *buzz*, are produced by adjusting the larynx so that it is phonating and providing an air flow that will generate noise at the constriction that the speaker forms near his teeth. Sounds like [z] are often considered to be both voiced and "strident" by phonologists who want to maintain binary distinctions in their description of the sounds of speech (Jakobson, Fant and Halle, 1963).

Interactions of the supralaryngeal vocal tract on fundamental frequency

The source–filter theory of speech production is generally interpreted to mean that the source and filter are completely independent factors. This is not really the case. The output of the larynx during phonation is affected by the

---

[3] Think of a crowd of people moving through a narrow passage from a large room; they will be moving faster in the narrow passageway. They would have to move still faster to maintain the same "rate of emptying" if they had to exit through a still narrower passageway. "Noise" would be generated as the people collided when they moved faster and faster.

supralaryngeal vocal tract. Interactions that affect the glottal waveform can be seen when the first formant frequency is low (Fant, 1960). These interactions may extend to changes in the fundamental frequency of phonation. Vowels that have a low first formant frequency tend to have higher fundamental frequencies, all other things being equal. The data of Peterson and Barney (1952), which were derived for speakers producing isolated words, and Shadle (1985) for fluent speech show that f_0 is about 10 Hz higher for /i/s and /u/s which have a low F_1, and 10 Hz lower for /a/s which have a high F_1. Some computational models of the larynx predict that this effect follows from aerodynamic coupling of the larynx and the supralaryngeal vocal tract (Flanagan *et al.*, 1970; Atkinson, 1973). However, other studies claim that these effects follow from muscular and postural interactions between supralaryngeal vocal tract articulatory maneuvers and the larynx (Ohala, 1970).

Aerostatic coupling between the larynx and the supralaryngeal vocal tract also takes place. Whenever the supralaryngeal vocal tract is obstructed, there must be a build-up in buccal (mouth) air pressure. Since the larynx is powered by the differential between the air pressure beneath and above it, the *transglottal air pressure, f_0,* will fall when, for example, a stop like [b] is produced in intervocalic position. The fundamental frequency will fall until the transglottal air pressure falls to about 2 cm H_2O when phonation stops. The aerodynamic and aerostatic coupling between the larynx and the supralaryngeal vocal tract will induce fluctuations in f_0 that are a consequence of the inherent physiological properties of the larynx. This has obvious implications for phonetic theories that attach linguistic significance to the small variations in fundamental frequency that continually occur during normal speech production.

The supralaryngeal vocal tract

As we demonstrated in Chapter 4, formant frequencies are determined by the cross-sectional area function of the supralaryngeal vocal tract. In Figure 6.12, the adult human vocal tract is sketched in a stylized midsagittal section. Some of the principal landmarks are noted on the sketch. The lips are, of course, evident. The nasal cavity, which is quite large, is isolated from the oral cavity by the palate and velum. The palate, which forms the roof of the mouth, consists of two parts. The anterior (front) hard palate consists of bone. The *velum* or soft palate is the posterior (rear) section of the palate. The velum is made up of muscles and soft tissue. When you breathe through your nose it falls downwards and frontwards, connecting the nasal cavity to the pharynx and larynx. During the production of speech it can move upwards and stiffen

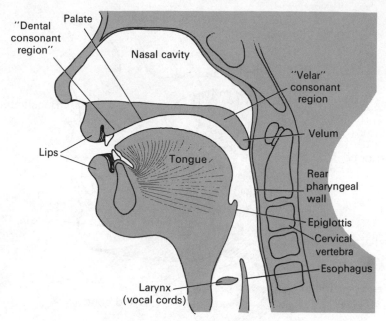

Figure 6.12. Stylized midsagittal section of adult human vocal tract.

to seal the nasal cavity from the oral cavity when these muscles tense. Table 6.1 notes how two of these muscles, the *levator palatini* and *palatoglossus*, can work. Figure 6.13 shows the position of the levator palatini (cf. tensor veli palatini).

The tongue, which mainly consists of a group of muscles, has a shape that is anatomically unique to modern *Homo sapiens*. In all other mammals the tongue is long and thin and is positioned entirely within the oral cavity (Negus, 1949). In human beings the posterior section of the tongue has a round contour in the midsagittal plane (Nearey, 1978) and forms both the lower surface of the oral cavity and the anterior margin of the pharynx. The unique geometry of the human supralaryngeal vocal tract evolved in the last 1.5 million years and, as we shall see, structures both the production and the perception of human speech (Lieberman, 1968, 1973, 1975, 1984; Lieberman and Crelin 1971; Laitman and Heimbuch, 1982). The rear pharyngeal wall is positioned in front of the *cervical vertebrae* of the spinal column which are sketched in Figure 6.12.

The human pharynx connects to the larynx which can be seen in the sketch in Figure 6.12. The open tube that is posterior to the larynx in Figure 6.12 is the entrance to the *esophagus*. The esophagus connects to the stomach. It is normally collapsed unless something is being swallowed. Humans are unique among terrestrial animals in this arrangement where the pharynx is a common

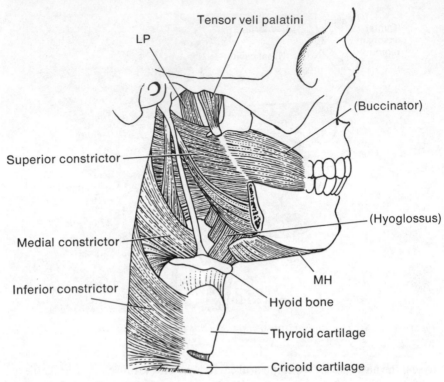

Figure 6.13. The pharyngeal constrictor muscles.

pathway for the ingestion of liquids and solid food which must be shunted into the esophagus, and for air which must enter the larynx. As Darwin (1859, p.191) noted, we are more susceptible to choking on food when we swallow than other animals. We have to propel food into the esophagus and keep it out of the larynx when we swallow. The larynx is therefore pulled upwards and forwards by tensioning the anterior body of the *digastric* muscle, while the pharyngeal constrictor muscles propel the food into the opened esophagus. Swallowing is a good example of a "programmed" act in which a complex series of motor acts proceed in a sequence of which the user is not consciously aware (Bosma, 1957). The muscles that are active during swallowing are also used for very different purposes in different patterns of activity in speech production. The process of "learning" to speak involves setting up new patterns of programmed activity.

In Figure 6.13 the pharyngeal constrictor muscles, some of the muscles of the soft palate and the cheek muscles (the *buccinators*), are sketched. The *superior constrictor* (SC), *medial constrictor* (MC), and *inferior constrictor* of

116

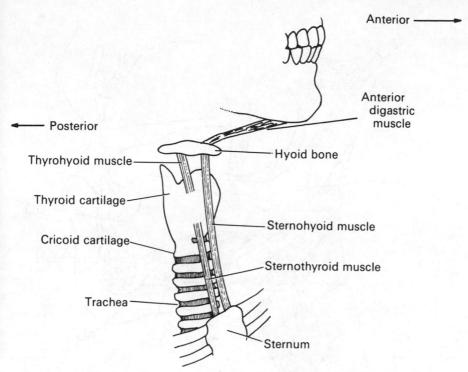

Figure 6.14. The "strap" muscles that connect the mandible, skull, larynx, and breastbone.

the pharynx propel food down the pharynx as they contract, one after the other. The *styloglossus* muscle (see Figure 6.15) runs from the styloid process of the temporal bone of the skull. We will discuss the muscles that are inserted (i.e. attached) to the styloid process a little later.

Muscles are often named by noting the bones, cartilages, or major soft tissue structures that they connect. This convention is useful in that it allows you to know that anatomical structures *could* be moved by the muscle. However, unless you know the total coordinated pattern of muscular activity of *all* the muscles that can affect these anatomical structures, you cannot predict what will happen when an individual muscle is activated. For example, the sternohyoid muscle (Figure 6.14) is activated when a person pulls the hyoid bone down. It also can be activated in conjunction with the anterior digastric to open the *mandible* (lower jaw), in which case the mandible pivots open while the hyoid stays put. All of the muscles that we will sketch and discuss are noted in Table 6.1, which is keyed to these diagrams. The "strap" muscles that connect the larynx to the mandible, skull, and *sternum* (breastbone), some of which have already been discussed, are sketched in Figure 6.14, while the

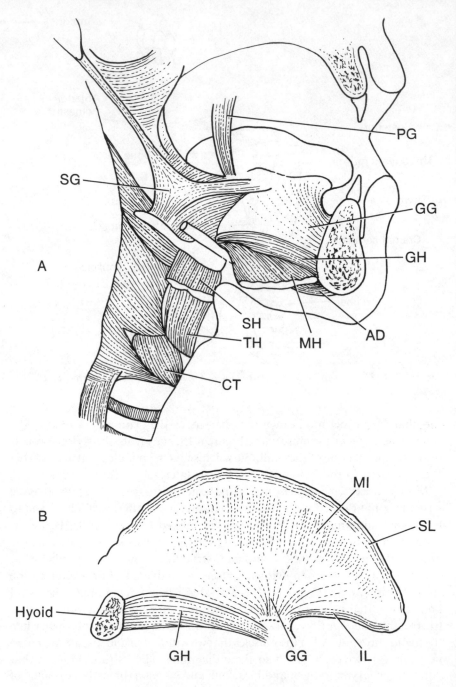

Figure 6.15. Some of the muscles of the tongue. See Table 6.1.

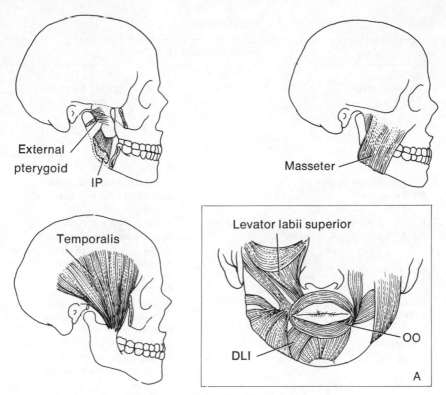

Figure 6.16. Muscles of the face and jaw. See Table 6.1.

muscles of the tongue and suprahyoid muscles are sketched in Figure 6.15. Some of the muscles of the face and the muscles that close and move the jaw are sketched in Figure 6.16.

Table 6.1 is not a comprehensive list of all of the muscles that can be involved in speech production. There is no general agreement on the function or functions of many of these muscles. It is apparent that different speakers use their muscles differently when they produce the "same" sounds. It is also apparent that these muscles are developed to a greater or lesser degree in different individuals. A more detailed listing of muscles and their possible activity may be found in Zemlin (1968).

Electromyographic studies of supralaryngeal muscles

These sketches do not show all of the muscles that can function during respiration, swallowing, chewing, or speaking. These muscles and those that close and open the lips, however, constitute most of the muscles that appear to

119

Table 6.1. *The muscles of speech production.*

Muscle	Figure reference	Function
A. Intrinsic	Larynx	
1. Thyroarytenoid (TA)	6.4	Vocal cord tensor, forms body of vocal cord; is active during f_0 change. Acts to change thickness of vocal cord for register changes; may also act to change overall tension of vocal cord for phonation in different registers.
2. Posterior circoarytenoid (PCA)	6.4	Opens the glottis for either breathing or the production of − *voiced* sounds.
3. Lateral cricoarytenoid (LCA)	6.4	Adducts the vocal cords; applies medial compression; is active during f_0 changes, always active in onset of phonation, when it adducts vocal cords, setting phonation neutral position.
4. Cricothyroid (CT)	6.4 6.15	Applies longitudinal tension to vocal cords; is active during f_0 changes.
5. Interarytenoid	—	Adducts the vocal cords; applies medial compression. May be active in setting phonation neutral position.
B. Extrinsic		
1. Sternohyoid (SH)	6.14 6.15	Lowers the hyoid *if* muscles that go from hyoid to skull and mandible are slack. Also stabilizes hyoid when muscles like digastric tense to open mandible. May be active in initiating phonation register shifts.
2. Thyrohyoid (TH)	6.14 6.15	Decreases distance between thyroid cartilage and hyoid bone.
3. Sternothyroid (ST)	6.14	Lowers the thyroid cartilage.
	Pharynx	
1. Superior constrictor (SC)	6.13	Constrict the pharynx; active during swallowing and in the
2. Medial constrictor (MC)	6.13	production of sounds like the vowel [a].
3. Inferior constrictor (IC)	6.13	
4. Palatopharyngeus	6.13	Constricts the pharynx; also can lower the soft palate.
	Soft palate	
1. Levator palatini	6.13	Raises soft palate, sealing nasal

Table 6.1. (*cont.*)

Muscle	Figure reference	Function
		cavity in the production of oral sounds. The SC also is active in some speakers when they seal their nasal cavity.
2. Palatoglossus (PG)	6.15	Raises tongue body or lowers soft palate.
	Tongue	
A. Intrinsic		
1. Superior longitudinal (SL)	6.15B	Turns up the tip of tongue.
2. Inferior longitudinal (IL)		Turns down the tip of tongue.
3. Transverse (MI)*	6.15B	Narrows the tip of tongue.
4. Vertical (MI)*	6.15B	Flattens the tip of tongue.
B. Extrinsic		
1. Genioglossus (GC)	6.15	Pulls tongue body forward; depresses the tongue body; can elevate the hyoid. Is active in production of sounds like [i] or [u], where pharynx is widened by tongue body moving forward.
2. Styloglossus	6.15	Pulls tongue body towards styloid process. Is probably active in production of sounds like [u] and velar consonants.
	Suprahyoid	
1. Anterior belly of digastric (AD)	6.14 6.15	Opens the jaw *if* the hyoid is stabilized by tensioning muscles that connect hyoid to sternum; raises hyoid otherwise. Can be used in the production of sounds like [a].
2. Geniohyoid (GH)	6.15	Opens jaw if hyoid is stabilized; raises hyoid and pulls it forward.
3. Mylohyoid (MH)	6.13 6.14 6.15	Raises tongue body.
	Mandible (lower jaw)	
1. Masseter (MAS)	6.16	Closes the jaw.
2. Temporalis (TEM)	6.16	Closes the jaw; pulls lower jaw backwards.

Table 6.1. (*cont.*)

Muscle	Figure reference	Function
3. Internal pterygoid (IP)	6.16	Closes the jaw.
	Lips and face	
1. Orbicularis oris (OO)	6.16A	Closes the mouth; puckers the lips; acts to close and round lips in sounds like [u].
2. Depressor labii inferior (DLI)		Opens and retracts lips. Active in the release of sounds like [p] and [b].
3. Levator labii superior		Opens lips; sometimes active in release of sounds like [p] and [b].

*MI includes both transverse and vertical.

play a part in the production of speech. We have not included sketches of some of the smaller muscles like the palatoglossus, which runs between the soft palate and the tongue, but these diagrams should provide sufficient orientation for the reader to follow discussions of muscle activity in papers reporting current research.

The patterns of muscular activity for different speakers are often quite different even when the speakers are producing the "same" sound in their native language. For example, the patterns of muscular activity for a "simple" act like sealing the nasal cavity from the oral cavity in the production of stop nasal clusters like those of the nonsense words [fipmip], [futmup], etc., varies for different speakers. Bell-Berti (1973) in a detailed electromyographic study of velopharyngeal closure found that the muscle control patterns of the three speakers she studied were very different. Two speakers consistently used their superior pharyngeal constrictors to help seal their nasal cavities during the production of the "oral" nonnasal stops [p], [t]. The third speaker presented almost no activity in either the superior constrictor or middle constrictor muscles that could be identified with oral articulation. Electromyographic studies of the oral versus nasal distinction have shown that one particular muscle, the *levator palatini*, is consistently associated with the production of this distinction (Lubker, Fritzell and Lindquist, 1970). When the levator palatini tenses it tends to seal the nasal cavity. Other muscles of the supralaryngeal vocal tract, however, act in concert with this muscle, but they do not behave as consistently. Different speakers exhibit different patterns of activity.

These data are not consistent with traditional phonetic theories or strong versions of the "motor theory of speech perception" which claim that invariant articulatory gestures or motor commands underlie the sounds of speech (Liberman *et al.*, 1967; Chomsky and Halle, 1968; Liberman and Mattingly, 1985). Electromyographic and quantitative articulatory studies show that different speakers of the same dialect produce the same speech sounds using different patterns of muscular activity. The speakers act as though they are trying to preserve *acoustic* distinctions by using different patterns of articulatory activity in different circumstances.

The following data may exemplify the different claims of phonetic theories based on *articulatory or motor invariance* versus theories based on *acoustic invariance*. These theories all aim at characterizing the physiology of speech production in a psychologically and linguistically meaningful way. We will discuss phonetic theories in more detail in Chapter 8 after we address the issues of speech perception, but it is appropriate to start the discussion here in relation to speech production. Traditional phonetic theories, which only date back to Bell's work in the mid nineteenth century, claim that a particular muscle command or articulatory gesture *always* stands in a one-to-one relationship with some linguistically significant speech distinction. Perhaps the simplest example is the binary *oral* versus *nasal* sound contrast (Chomsky and Halle, 1968). Phonological evidence from many human languages demonstrates that speech sounds can differ in a linguistically significant way in a *binary* mode for this distinction (Jakobson, Fant and Halle, 1963). A sound like the English consonant [m] thus differs minimally from [b] in that [m] is nasalized. This minimal distinction is *phonological* because it can be used to differentiate words in English, e.g. *mat* versus *bat*. This phonological sound contrast superficially appears to be based on an invariant articulatory motor command. Electromyographic data show that the *levator palatini* muscle always contracts when a speaker produces an oral sound, e.g. the English stop [b]. The binary *oral* versus *nasal* sound contrast thus seemingly could be directly related to the activity of this particular muscle. If the speaker tensions his levator palatini muscle, the sound will be oral. If he does not tension this muscle, the sound will be nasal. The distinction would be a binary one + *levator palatini tensioning* versus − *levator palatini tensioning*. However, this classificatory scheme will not work because a speaker may use varying degrees of levator palatini activity in producing different oral sounds, and sometimes will even produce "oral" sounds without tensing this muscle.

The aerodynamic phenomena that determine the degree of "coupling" between the nasal cavity and the velopharyngeal port (the region of the supralaryngeal vocal tract where the velum and pharynx meet, cf. Figure 6.12) depend on the nature of the sound that is being formed in the supralaryngeal vocal tract. The vowels [i] and [u] (in *meet* and *boot*) require a tighter velopharyngeal port seal than the vowel [a] (the first vowel of *father*) when they are produced as [−*nasal*] vowels (House and Stevens, 1956). The three speakers of English monitored by Bell-Berti (1973) consistently used more levator palatini activity for these vowels. In other words, the speakers used more muscle activity to effect a tighter seal of the nasal cavity when it was necessary to do this to produce the desired signal. The elevation of the velum (the soft palate) began earlier and achieved a greater peak magnitude for the vowels [i] and [u] than for [a]. These speakers, in fact, did not bother to raise their velums for the vowel [a] after nasal consonants where the slight nasal quality was not very evident at the acoustic level. The common phonetic distinction between the nasalized and oral vowel pairs [a] versus [ã], [i] versus [ĩ], and [u] versus [ũ] (where the symbol ˜ indicates nasality) is the presence of the formants and "zeros" that are the acoustic correlates of nasality (Fant, 1960; Fujimura, 1962). The activity of the muscles that generate these acoustic correlates vary for the different vowels, even when we restrict our attention to a single speaker.

Electromyographic studies also demonstrate that it is impossible to associate any particular muscle with a unique sound contrast. Although the levator palatini muscle is closely associated with the nasal-versus-oral sound contrast, it also enters into the control of phonation in the production of stop consonants like [b] (Yanagihara and Hyde, 1966). The pharyngeal constrictors are also active in the production of the differences in anterioposterior width that enter into the production of sounds like vowels [i], [u], and [a].

Cineradiographic studies

In Figure 6.17 a diagram is reproduced of a frame from an X-ray movie of the vocal tract of an adult speaker during the production of speech. The diagram is a reproduction of a tracing of a single frame of this movie. The subject was positioned in front of an image-intensifying apparatus that permits X-ray views to be made with reduced levels of exposure. The tracing was part of a quantitative study (Perkell, 1969) in which measurements of the displacements of various parts of the vocal tract were made for every frame of a slow motion, sound-synchronized cineradiograph of a single adult speaker (Professor Kenneth N. Stevens of the Massachusetts Institute of Technology) carefully pronouncing a list of short syllables. The cineradiographic film was specially processed to enhance its quality. The subject's head was stabilized while he spoke and lead pellets were glued to his tongue to serve as reference points. The film's frames were numbered and measured and compared with sound spectrograms. In short, great effort was expended towards enhancing

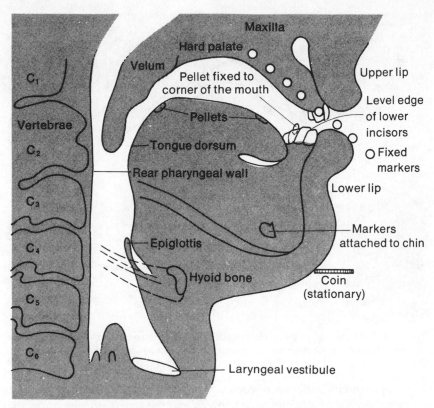

Figure 6.17. Diagram of a frame from an X-ray movie of the vocal tract of an adult human male during the production of speech. Anatomical features are labeled. Reprinted from Physiology of speech production *by Joseph Perkell, by permission of the MIT Press, Cambridge, Mass. Copyright 1969.*

accuracy. In Figure 6.18 the midline contour of the tongue is sketched for the different vowels that occurred in this cineradiographic study. Note that the pharyngeal anterioposterior width of [a] is narrowest. The pharyngeal constrictor muscles tense, narrowing the pharynx in the production of an [a]. The pharynx is narrowed laterally as well as in its anterioposterior dimension. Changes in the lateral dimension of the pharynx do not show up in radiographs like that sketched in Figure 6.18 but they have been monitored by using pulsed ultrasound (a technique similar to the use of sonar to locate the ocean floor). Movements of up to 5 millimetres of the lateral pharyngeal wall occur in the production of an [a]. There is little or no movement of the lateral pharyngeal wall in the production of an [i] or [u] (Minifie *et al.*, 1970).

The sketches of the tongue contour for each vowel that are presented in Figure 6.18 represent the most extreme movement of the tongue for each vowel

125

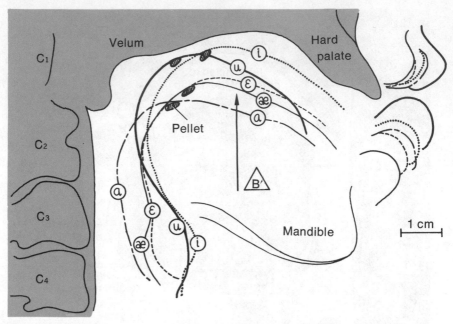

Figure 6.18. Midline contours of the tongue for the same speaker as shown in Figure 6.17. Reprinted from Physiology of speech production *by Joseph Perkell, by permission of the MIT Press, Cambridge, Mass. Copyright 1969.*

at the approximate midpoint of each vowel. The tongue is constantly moving during the production of connected speech and the articulatory gestures that correspond to individual segments of speech are "melded" together (Daniloff and Moll, 1968; MacNeilage and DeClerk, 1969; MacNeilage, 1970) as is the acoustic signal (Ohman, 1966; Liberman *et al.*, 1967). It is possible to describe the process of speech production in terms of individual segments that are "coarticulated." The effect of a segment on the segments that occur before it can be viewed as "anticipatory coarticulation." Thus the position of the tongue in the production of the sound [t] in the word *tale* differs from the position for the [t] in the word *tile*. The position of the tongue in the production of the sound [l] likewise will differ in these two words because of "post coarticulation" effects. The effects of each "segment" on other "segments" of speech is, however, so pervasive that it is more realistic to view the movements of the articulatory apparatus as "encoded" sequences that encompass at least one syllable (Gay, 1974; Nearey, 1976; Lieberman, 1976).

Cineradiographic data also demonstrate that the articulatory maneuvers that underlie speech are different between speakers of the same dialect when they produce the "same" sound, and that the particular articulatory maneuvers do not correspond with the hypothetical articulatory gestures that structure traditional phonetic theories (Houde, 1967; Perkell, 1969; Ladefoged *et al.*, 1972; Nearey, 1978). Cineradiographic studies consistently show that the movements of individual articulators are affected by the preceding and following speech sounds (Gay, 1974). New radiographic techniques have been devised that make use of a computer and a "microbeam" that illuminates only a small area (Fujimura, Tatsumi and Kagaya, 1973; Abbs, 1986). The X-ray dosage to the subject can be kept at or under the level that follows from natural sources in a normal environment. These techniques will allow speech scientists to obtain repeated measurements of speech production without undue medical hazards. It is clear that we need more data that address issues like variation and the dynamic control of fluent speech.

Automatization, coarticulation, and planning

As we noted earlier, monitoring the activity of a single isolated muscle is insufficient to characterize the production of a speech sound. It is necessary, therefore, to consider the activity of functionally related muscles when we study the production of speech (Abbs, 1986; Tuller and Kelso, 1984). The linguistic, i.e. meaningful, distinctions between the sounds of speech derive from the coordinated activity of many muscles operating in close synchrony. Some studies claim that articulatory coordination is maintained by means of mechanical principles similar to those that determine the frequency at which a mass supported by a spring will vibrate after it has been displaced from its equilibrium point (Tuller and Kelso, 1984; Fowler and Smith, 1985). These mechanical principles are, to cite a more familiar example, similar to those which determine the frequency at which a car will bounce after you push down on its bumper. The complex pattern of coordinated activity that we observe in the production of speech is supposed to follow from the mechanical properties of the speech production anatomy – without any other goal-directed neural planning.

Though this issue is contested, a number of studies demonstrate that there is more to speech production than this. Speech production appears to involve what Folkins (1985) terms an "integrated motor approach." Folkins (1985) reviews the results of many experiments that indicate that the speaker's goal is to produce an acoustic output that is perceptually appropriate. Human speakers rapidly execute complex articulatory patterns to achieve particular acoustic goals. These articulatory patterns appear to be produced by means of the neural process of *automatization* (Lieberman, 1973, 1975). Though human beings appear to have evolved neural mechanisms that are specialized for the automatization of the articulatory maneuvers that underlie speech (Lieberman, 1984), the general process of automatization is not limited to the production of speech. Automatization (Evarts, 1973) is the process which allows animals to rapidly execute complex goal-directed patterns of motor activity. Most of the "learned" routines of our daily lives as well as those of other species are automatized (MacClean, 1985). An experienced car driver shifts gears using an automatized sequence – a rapid pattern of motor activity that is executed without conscious thought. The motor activity that character-izes much of our life is "routine" and "automatic" because it is executed by means of reflex-like neural subroutines that execute goal-directed activity. Automatization yields quick responses to external stimuli in the absence of specific innate mechanisms shaped to every possible contingency, such as the innate mechanisms that determine the response patterns of bullfrogs (Lettvin *et al.*, 1959). Automatization also allows an animal to focus on the "creative," higher level aspects of a task, whether it involves driving a car, playing a piano concerto, speaking, or stalking a mouse. There is an obvious selective advantage for the enhancement of the neural bases of automatization at every level of animal life.

Electrophysiological data (e.g. Evarts, 1973; Polit and Bizzi, 1978; Miles and Evarts, 1979) demonstrate that the acquisition of automatized motor activity involves the formation of a direct, reflex-like control loop in the motor cortex in which afferent input from muscle spindles initiates a response in neurons that direct motor activity towards particular goals. Evarts, for example, trained a monkey to grasp a movable handle and position it in a particular area on a target. An external force then abruptly moved the handle out of the correct area. The monkey would gain a reward by promptly returning the handle to the correct area. Using microelectrode techniques, recordings were made from the hand area of the monkey's motor cortex. Responses in neurons in this area of the motor cortex occurred 24 milliseconds after the handle was perturbed. The muscles of the monkey's arm registered EMG signals 7 milliseconds after these cortical neurons responded. The total time delay from the presentation of the perturbing force to the corrective muscle activity in the monkey's arm was about 40 milliseconds, about twice as fast as the response times typical of cross-modal, e.g. visual to motor, feedback. These response patterns were absent in untrained monkeys. The conclusion reached by Evarts is that the trained monkey's motor responses in this task were controlled by a pathway through the motor cortex that had been acquired and that was goal-directed. The goal coded in an automatized motor cortex pathway may be a simple one – resisting the deflection of one's forearm by external forces – or complex – producing the formant frequency patterns of the sound [b]. However, the essential aspect of automatization is that a complex motor routine that may involve the activity of different muscles is neurally coded and executed as a subroutine, directed to a functional goal.

A number of recent studies of the production of speech in normal speakers suggest that speech production appears to involve the speaker's planning his articulatory maneuvers to achieve supralaryngeal vocal tract shapes that yield particular *acoustic* goals. These studies make use of artificial impediments and "perturbations" to the production of speech to determine what the speaker is aiming to produce. Folkins and Zimmerman (1981), for example, show that the muscular activity of speakers producing utterances while their jaws are constrained by *bite-blocks* appears to involve automatized motor patterns. A bite-block is a device that the speaker clenches between his teeth as he talks. The bite-block can be made of a small piece of wood or dental material with a string attached to it to prevent the speaker from accidentally swallowing it. Folkins and Zimmerman monitored motion of the speaker's jaw as well as the electrical activity of the muscles that close the mandible, the masseter and internal pterygoid muscles (c.f. Table 6.1 and Figure 6.16). Four normal adult speakers were monitored during the production of repeated sequences of the syllables [pæ] and [pɪ] under a normal condition and when bite-blocks were inserted between the subjects' upper and lower molar teeth. In one bite-block condition there was a 5 mm gap between the subjects' central incisor teeth; the second bite-block condition resulted in a 15 mm gap. The subjects compensated for the bite-blocks by appropriate adjustments in their tongue and lip movements. For example, they moved their tongues further in the bite-block conditions when they produced the syllable [pɪ] to produce the same acoustic signal that occurred in the normal control condition. However, there was no difference in the timing or magnitude of the activity of the muscles that they would have used to close their jaws, when their jaws were fixed by the bite-blocks. The automatized muscle commands for the production of these syllables were activated, even though they knew and could feel that their jaws could not move. The speakers added compensatory tongue and lip movements to generate the acoustic signal but did not modify the basic automatized motor control pattern that is adjusted to the normal requirements of speech production in which the speaker closes his jaw.

The results of many bite-block experiments (Lindblom, Lubker and Gay, 1979) suggest that speakers have some sort of mental representation of the supralaryngeal vocal tract shape that they normally use to produce a particular speech sound in a given phonetic context. Bite-block induced deviations from the normal conditions result in the speakers' producing the appropriate supralaryngeal vocal tract shape by means of compensating motor activity, i.e. by moving their tongue and lips to compensate for their fixed mandibles. These compensatory maneuvers take place within milliseconds after the speaker starts to produce the sound, excluding the possibility of the speaker monitoring the sound first auditorily and then executing compensatory motor commands.

Experiments that make use of rapid perturbations of the vocal apparatus show that speakers have access to different patterns of automatized motor control that share a common goal – producing an acceptable acoustic signal. The proper execution of the bilabial stop consonant [b], for example, involves a speaker's momentarily occluding the supralaryngeal airway with his lips. Gracco and Abbs (1985) in an articulatory perturbation experiment used a small torque motor that applied a force to a speaker's lower lip. The speakers in this experiment were producing a series of syllables that started with the consonant [b]. The experimenters first used the motor to apply a force to the speaker's lower lip 40 milliseconds before the point in time that the lips would normally reach a closed position. The perturbing force would have prevented the proper execution of the bilabial stop consonant [b]. However, the speaker compensated by applying more force to his lower lip to overcome the perturbing force; the speaker also applied a slight downwards movement of his upper lip. The experimenters then applied the perturbing force 20 milliseconds before the normal lip closure. The speaker in this case compensated by a large downwards movement of his upper lip, extending the duration of the lip closure gesture. The speaker, in other words, used two different automatized motor patterns that had a common goal – closing the lips to produce the consonantal stop closure. The compensating motor activity for both perturbation conditions occurred within 40 milliseconds, far too short a time interval for cross-modal auditory feedback. The compensating activity must be initiated by afferent signals from the perturbed lip to the motor cortex and effected by control signals directly from the motor cortex. The compensating action involves goal-directed activity which can be effected by different patterns of muscular activity. The same speaker under different timing conditions compensates by mainly increasing the activity of his lower lip – moving it upwards – or by mainly moving his upper lip downwards. The speaker appears to have a neural representation in the motor cortex of an abstract linguistic *goal*, closing one's lips for a [b].

The genesis of the automatized motor control patterns that appear to underlie the production of human speech is unclear. It is unlikely that all of these motor patterns are innate, i.e. genetically transmitted in *Homo sapiens*. The data of Lubker and Gay (1982), for example, show that adult speakers of Swedish and American English have different patterns when they coarticulate *lip-rounding*. One of the articulatory gestures that is essential for the production of the vowel [u] is lip-rounding (Stevens and House, 1955). The speaker protrudes and purses the lips. Lubker and Gay monitored the electrical activity of eight native speakers of Swedish and American English in an experiment on *anticipatory*, i.e. *pre-planned*, coarticulation. It had been previously observed that speakers rounded their lips when a consonant like [t] preceded an [u]. It is unnecessary to round one's lips in producing a [t], but it does not affect the acoustic correlates that specify a [t] if you do round your lips. Thus speakers can optionally plan ahead, rounding their lips for the vowel [u] that they "know" will come. Lubker and Gay found different temporal patterns for native speakers of Swedish and American English, as well as some individual differences among the speakers of Swedish. In the production of syllables in a consonant like [t] preceding an [u], speakers of American English start to round their lips about 100 milliseconds before the start of phonation for the vowel. The American English speaker will not start to lip-round earlier even if several other consonants intercede between the [t] and the [u]. In contrast, some speakers of Swedish will start to round 500 milliseconds in advance of the [u]. Other speakers of Swedish used time intervals that were intermediate between 100 and 500 milliseconds. It is most unlikely that a systematic genetic difference could account for these differences. Rather, the speakers of the two languages probably learn automatized motor patterns as they acquire their native language. The process of speech acquisition by children, which we shall discuss in Chapter 9, is likely to involve the gradual acquisition of these automatized motor patterns (Lieberman, 1984).

Not all of the distinctions that occur in speech production are strictly "linguistic." Children learn to specify their intended *gender* by means of automatized speech motor commands. One of the characteristics of a person that is transmitted by the speech signal is the intended gender of the person, i.e. whether that person intends to be perceived as male or female. Our "intuition" tells us that gender is transmitted by the average perceived pitch of the person's voice, which is closely related to the fundamental frequency of phonation (Flanagan, 1972). However, our intuitions in this matter are wrong, at least for speakers of American English. There is considerable overlap in the average fundamental frequencies of phonation for adult male and female speakers (Lieberman, 1967). Furthermore, we know that young boys and girls have about the same fundamental frequencies (Robb and Saxman, 1985). However, a study of five-year-old children shows that with the exception of a few "tomboys," girls' and boys' voices can be sorted for gender (Sachs, Lieberman and Erikson, 1972). The boys turn out to be producing speech sounds that have lower average formant frequencies than girls. This difference does not follow from their supralaryngeal vocal tract anatomy. Children at this age have roughly the same anatomy except for primary sexual differences. There is no consistent difference in height, weight, etc. until the onset of puberty (Crelin, 1973). What the boys do is to automatize a set of speech motor patterns in which they round their lips to drive their formant frequencies lower. They are modeling their behavior on the average difference that exists between adult males and females. Adult males, on average, are larger than females and have longer supralaryngeal vocal tracts (Fant, 1966). But this group difference does

131

not necessarily typify an individual who wants to sound male. Boys and many adult men who have short supralaryngeal vocal tracts therefore learn to round their lips and execute other articulatory maneuvers that yield lower formant frequencies (Mattingly, personal communication; Goldstein, 1980). It is difficult to shift the average fundamental frequency of one's voice without causing laryngeal pathologies (Kirchner, 1970), so gender is conveyed by learned automatized supralaryngeal vocal tract maneuvers that shift formant frequencies.

Supralaryngeal vocal tract modeling

In Chapter 4 we calculated the formant frequencies for supralaryngeal vocal tract area functions that approximate uniform tubes. The formant frequencies of more complex supralaryngeal vocal tract area functions can be determined by various techniques. The simplest technique, in principle, is to construct a mechanical model of the supralaryngeal vocal tract and then excite it by means of appropriate acoustic sources. If we know the area function we can make a tube by hammering it out of brass, molding plastic, machining plastics, etc. If the area function that we are modeling is a vowel that is normally excited by a glottal source, we can place an artificial larynx at the glottal end and measure the formant frequencies of the sound that the tube produces. The transfer functions of consonants excited by noise generated at the constriction can be determined by passing air through the model. The material that is used to make the walls of the mechanical model does not have to match the sound absorbing and transmitting characteristics of the human supralaryngeal vocal tract since appropriate corrections can be made to compensate for such differences (Fant, 1960). Mechanical models are particularly useful for simulating and analyzing the nonlinear effects that are associated with the sound sources of [voiced] sounds. A schematic of a model and the techniques for making acoustic measurements is shown in Figure 6.19. The model makes it possible to assess the significance of the articulatory maneuvers that can be observed in cineradiographic data. It would be difficult otherwise to determine the acoustic consequences of different variations in the articulation of this sound.

The data that we can derive from a lateral X-ray are insufficient if we want to determine the acoustic consequences of articulatory maneuvers. The transfer function of the supralaryngeal vocal tract is a function of the cross-sectional area function. It is therefore necessary to derive an area function from the X-ray view. This is quite a difficult task. The experimenter must make use of whatever data are available. Dental casts of the oral cavity, photographs of the lips, X-ray views from the front, measurements from cadavers, and ultrasonic scans all are useful (Chiba and Kajiyama, 1941; Fant, 1960; Heinz, 1962; Goldstein, 1980).

132

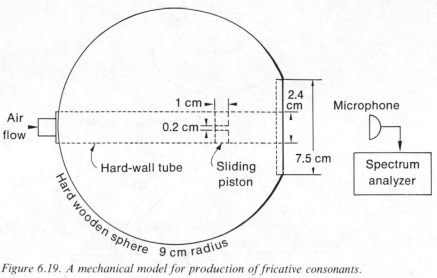

Figure 6.19. A mechanical model for production of fricative consonants.

Analog models

Although it would be possible to use mechanical models of the vocal tract to determine the transfer function of any arbitrary area function, it is more convenient to use either analog or digital computer modeling techniques. The digital computer-implemented modeling technique is most frequently used today but it is useful to understand the principles of analog modeling which underlie most of the computer techniques.

Suppose that you were in charge of an agricultural water distribution system and wanted to determine how to regulate the flow of water into different fields. You could construct a simple analog model of the system. The analog principle that you could make use of is the similar mathematical relationship that holds between the electrical parameters of *voltage, current* and *resistance* and the hydraulic parameters of *pressure, flow* and *resistance*. In Figure 6.20 the water supply system is sketched. It consists of a reservoir, which may be more or less full depending on weather conditions, a main supply channel, two branch channels which go to the two fields in question, and two valves that can be set to introduce variable obstacles to the water flow into either field.

The problem is how to regulate the water flow as the height of the water in the reservoir changes. The electrical analog of Figure 6.21 would solve this problem. The resistance of the main supply channel is represented by the fixed electrical resistor R_s, the two branch channels are represented by the fixed resistors R_1 and R_2, respectively, and the two valves by the variable resistors VR_1 and VR_2. The voltage V is set by adjusting the control of a variable voltage source. The analog works by measuring (by means of simple meters) the

133

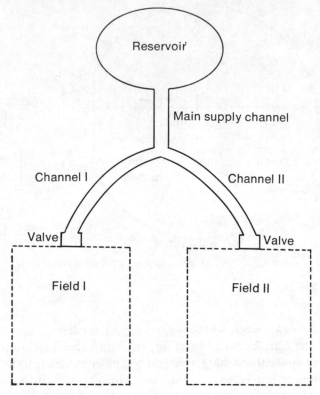

Figure 6.20. Sketch of water supply system.

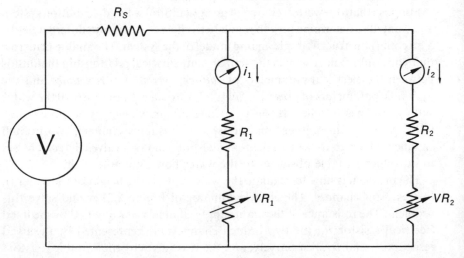

Figure 6.21. Electrical analog of water supply system.

electrical currents i_1 and i_2 that flow through the two branch circuits for particular values of V, VR_1 and VR_2. Voltage is analogous to water pressure and current to water flow because Ohm's law

$V = i(R)$

which describes the relationship between electrical current, voltage and resistance, also holds for the hydraulic variables,

pressure = flow (resistance)

The analog values appropriate for the resistors R_s, R_1 and R_2 can be determined by simple measurements once the system is set up. The usefulness of the analog system would become more apparent with more complex water distribution systems. It could be easily extended to very complex water distribution systems that had 50 or 100 channels.

The analog relationships that are appropriate for the construction of electrical analogs of the vocal tract involve relationships like that which hold between a force and the acceleration of matter, e.g. Newton's first law of motion and the voltage change across an inductor. (An inductor is an electrical device that can be constructed using a coil of wire.) The analog between Newton's first law of motion that applies to the acceleration of the air particles in the vocal tract and the voltage across the inductor is

$$F = m\frac{dv}{dt} \quad \text{Newton's first law of motion}$$

$$V = L\frac{di}{dt} \quad \text{Voltage across an inductor}$$

where dv/dt is the derivative of velocity with respect to time, F the force, and m the mass in Newton's law. The electrical analogs are V the voltage, L the inductance, and di/dt the derivative of the current with respect to time. Detailed discussions of electrical analogs like those contained in Flanagan (1972) are beyond the scope of this introduction. The essential point is that the principles of analog modeling are quite straightforward. The use of an analog model permits us to easily obtain quantitative measurements of variables that otherwise would be difficult or impossible to make.

"Terminal" analog studies of speech

Several phases or trends are apparent when the results of analog studies of the supralaryngeal vocal tract are reviewed. The first phase used "terminal" analysis and demonstrated that the source–filter theory was an adequate description of speech production. Electrical analogs that specified formants and antiformants were excited by glottal or noise sources to synthesize speech signals (Stevens, Kasouski and Fant, 1953; Fant, 1960). Psychoacoustic tests (which we will discuss in more detail in Chapter 7) demonstrated that human listeners perceived particular speech sounds if the appropriate formants and antiformants were specified. Since these synthesizers were designed by electrical engineers, the terminology of electrical circuit theory is often encountered in the research papers. The formant frequencies of the supralaryngeal vocal tract are essentially the frequencies at which a normal mode of vibration exists in the system. We illustrated this in Chapter 4 when we derived the formant frequencies of the uniform tube as the frequencies at which the physical system most readily supports a sinusoidal wave. This definition of the term *formant* is essentially that first proposed by Hermann (1894). It is equivalent to the way in which the term *pole* is used to characterize an electrical network (Stevens and House, 1961). The term *resonance* or *damped resonance* is often used to indicate the formants of a system.

The acoustic properties of the supralaryngeal vocal tract for unnasalized vowels, e.g. most of the vowels of English, involve only formants or poles, and they can thus be synthesized by "terminal analog" devices (Flanagan, 1957) that generate only formant frequencies. Sounds in which more than one airway is interposed between the source of acoustic energy and the outside environment, e.g. the nasalized vowels of Portuguese, also have an antiformant at which energy is absorbed. The term *zero* is used to designate this characteristic of an electrical network and is used to denote the antiformants of speech sounds (Fant, 1960; Fujimura, 1962). Consonants that are excited by sources located at points above the larynx typically have both formants and antiformants. The experimenter using a "terminal analog" need only specify the frequencies of the formants and antiformants (and their relative amplitudes if a "parallel" analog synthesizer is being used) (Lawrence, 1953; Stevens, Kasouski and Fant, 1953; Holmes, Mattingly and Shearme, 1964). In other words, the experimenters in theory do not need to know anything about the area function of the supralaryngeal vocal tract; they simply need to derive the formants and antiformants of the acoustic signal that they want to synthesize. Terminal synthesizers are usually implemented as computer software systems (Klatt, 1980) which can allow the experimenter to make fine adjustments in the parameters that may be relevant for the perception of a particular speech sound or class of sounds.

Area function analogs

Area function analogs of the supralaryngeal vocal tract model the vocal tract by using electrical networks that simulate the effect of changing vocal tract geometry. The first of these devices was constructed by Dunn (1950) and

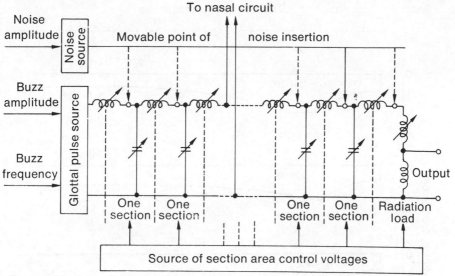

Figure 6.22. Controllable electrical vocal tract model. (After Rosen, 1958.)

represented the vocal tract as a series of sections each 0.5 centimetres long. A sketch of a controllable vocal tract analog which includes a "nose" nasal section is shown in Figure 6.22. The effective cross-sectional area of each section can be electrically adjusted. Devices like this analog (Stevens, Kasouski and Fant, 1953; Rosen, 1958; Fant, 1960) and more recent computer-implemented models (Henke, 1966; Flanagan *et al.*, 1970; Flanagan, Ishizaka and Shipley, 1975; Goldstein, 1980) permit experimenters to assess the acoustic significance of changes in the cross-sectional area of the supra-laryngeal vocal tract.

Stevens and House (1955) controlled the cross-sectional area of an electrical analog of the vocal tract by systematically varying the effects of lip protrusion and lip opening, and the position and degree of tongue constriction. The diagram in Figure 6.23, which shows some of the area functions that they modeled, indicates the parameters that they used to specify the shape of the vocal tract. Note that there is no nasal section, so the results are relevant for [−nasal] vowels. The distance from the glottis appears as the scale at the top of the figure. The radius of the supralaryngeal vocal tract tube appears as the vertical scale for the four vocal tract configurations sketched. The notations at the right specifying the A/l values represent A, the cross-sectional area of the lips, divided by l, the length of the lip passage.

The phonetic dimension of *lip-rounding* which we discussed earlier derives from the combined effects of lip protrusion and lip opening. These effects are combined into the single parameter A/l in this model for the reasons that we

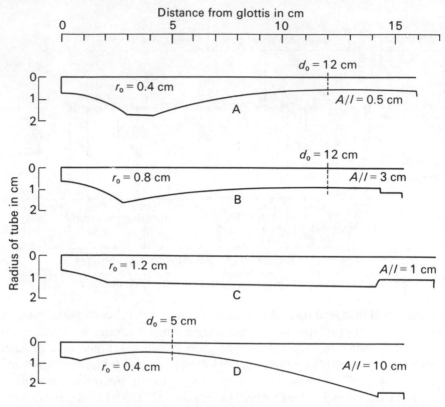

Figure 6.23. Vocal tract parameters controlled by Stevens and House (1955).

discussed in Chapter 4. A given value of A/l can be produced in different ways; for example, a mouth opening $A/l = 3$ cm could be achieved by a vocal tract shape of 1 cm long with $A = 3$ cm², or one that was 3 cm long with $A = 9$ cm². In either case the acoustic effect of the mouth opening would be approximately the same. The A/l values that Stevens and House used were derived from X-ray movies and high-speed movies of lip opening and varied from about 20 cm for the vowel [æ] to about 0.1 cm for [u]. The point of constriction of the vocal tract by the tongue body was specified by the number d_0, the distance of the most constricted part of the vocal tract from the glottis, and r_0, the radius at the constriction. The values of d_0 and r_0 were derived from X-ray data. The shape of the tongue was assumed to follow a parabolic function for all constrictions. There are some additional constraints on these control parameters that involve the effects of a large constriction near the glottis and the effects of the mandible and lips.

Supralaryngeal vocal tract modeling and phonetic theory

The Stevens and House modeling study demonstrates that it is possible to generate most vowels by means of very different area functions which may, or may not, correspond with shapes consistent with traditional phonetic theory. Different combinations of tongue position, tongue height, and A/l can produce identical acoustic signals. The only vowels that "require" particular area functions are [i], [u], and to a lesser extent, [a]. The values of F_1 and F_2 that specify a vowel like [ɪ] (the vowel in *bit*) in the Peterson and Barney formant frequency study (1952) can be produced by many different combinations of lip opening and rounding (as specified by the parameter A/l) and tongue position (the parameters d_0 and r_0). The Stevens and House modeling study thus suggests that acoustic factors may play a primary role in classifying vowel sounds. The auditory nature of traditional vowel diagrams has been discussed in many studies (Russell, 1928; Jones, 1932; Peterson, 1951; Jakobson, Fant and Halle, 1963; Ladefoged *et al.*, 1972); we will take stock of the controversy in Chapter 8. The question of the auditory versus the articulatory classification of vowels is part of the more general question of the physiological basis of phonetic theory.

Exercises

1. Compute the formant frequencies of an adult speaker having a 17 cm long supralaryngeal vocal tract (with his lips and larynx at rest) for the uniform tube configuration. The speaker's normal average fundamental frequency of phonation is 120 Hz. The speaker is in a space capsule in which the atmosphere is a mixture of helium and oxygen gases. The velocity of sound in this gas mixture is twice that of normal air.

    What will the formant frequencies of this speaker's [i] and [u] vowels be under these conditions? Explain the basis for your calculations.

    Compute the formant frequencies of a five-year-old child having a 8.5 cm long supralaryngeal vocal tract for the uniform tube configuration when the child is breathing normal air. This speaker's normal average fundamental frequency of phonation is 400 Hz.

2. Some studies in the 1950s claimed that each opening movement of the larynx was initiated by the contraction of a muscle. Subsequent studies found that this was not the case. How does the larynx produce phonation?

3. Linguists are in general agreement concerning the binary nature of "noise" excitation. A sound is either noise excited or it is not. Are the articulatory maneuvers that people use to generate noise "binary," all-or-nothing gestures? What physical phenomenon determines the binary nature of this linguistic contrast?

4. Explain speech "encoding."

7

Speech synthesis and speech perception

Vocoder synthesizers

The pace of research on the perception of speech corresponds in a meaningful way with the development of speech synthesizers. The initial impetus for work on speech synthesis was commercial. In the 1930s Dudley and his colleagues at Bell Telephone Laboratories developed the Vocoder (Dudley, 1936, 1939). The Vocoder is a device that first analyzes a speech signal by means of a set of electronic filters and a fundamental frequency extracting device. The electronic filters derive an approximation of the spectrum of the speech signal as a function of time while the fundamental frequency extractor simultaneously derives the fundamental frequency, or in the case of − *voiced* sounds indicates a noiselike source excitation. The electrical signals derived by the spectrum channels and the fundamental frequency extractor are then transmitted to a synthesizer in which the acoustic signal is reconstructed.

The diagram in Figure 7.1 illustrates a Vocoder system. The signal from the fundamental frequency extractor (the pitch channel) is used to drive a pulse generator (relaxation oscillator) in the Vocoder synthesizer. The output of the Vocoder synthesizer thus has the same periodicity as the input signal. The Vocoder was developed to serve as a speech transmission system that would reduce the frequency bandwidth that is necessary to transmit a speech signal. Although the Vocoder equipment might be expensive, it would more than pay for itself if it allowed the telephone company to "squeeze" twice as many messages into the frequency channel of a transoceanic telephone cable, for example. The frequency channel of any electronic transmission system is always subject to some finite limit. In the case of a transatlantic cable, the bandwidth of the channel is comparatively limited and the channel's cost is very great. Systems like the Vocoder thus were very attractive; if successful they would save millions of dollars. Vocoders, however, have never become widely accepted because the quality of the speech signal is degraded by the process of analysis and synthesis. The fundamental frequency extractors, in particular, do not work very well.

Dudley and his coworkers realized that the Vocoder's synthesizer could be

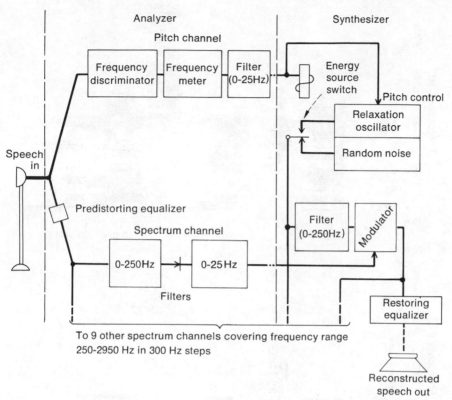

Figure 7.1. Vocoder block diagram. (After Dudley, 1936.)

used as a synthetic speaker (Dudley, Reisz and Watkins, 1939) by supplying artificially generated control signals in place of the signals that would have been derived by the analyzer. The synthesizer thus could be used to generate speechlike signals that, in fact, were never spoken. By precisely specifying the control signals, experimenters could systematically generate artificial speech signals and present these signals to human listeners, who could be asked to identify the signals and discriminate between slightly different versions of the signal, etc.

Various ingenious methods for controlling speech synthesizers derived from the Vocoder principle have been devised. Perhaps the most wide-ranging and seminal series of experiments came from the Haskins Laboratories group. A system was devised that would convert sound spectrograms or simplified sound spectrograms into acoustic signals (Cooper *et al.*, 1952). In Figure 7.2 a sound spectrogram made with a narrow-bandwidth filter (A) and a simplified tracing of the formant frequency patterns of the same spectrogram (B) are

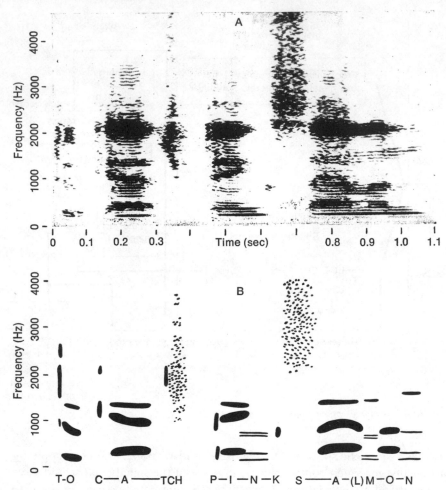

Figure 7.2. (A) Sound spectrogram. (B) Simplified version of the same phrase that serves as input to pattern playback. (After Cooper et al., 1952.)

presented. The formant frequencies which typically change as functions of time are represented as the dark areas on tracing B. The stippled areas represent noise excitation. The simplified spectrogram when converted to an acoustic signal is intelligible, although it does not sound very natural.

Speech synthesis and segmentation

The practical goal of the Haskins Laboratories group was to devise a machine that would "read aloud" to blind people. The machine was to identify

142

alphabetic characters in printed texts and convert these symbols into sounds that a blind person could listen to. It is not that difficult to devise a print-reading device, although this would not be necessary if the machine's use were to be restricted to the "reading" of new books and publications. At some stage in the preparation of a manuscript a machine with a keyboard is used. The talking machine could be connected to the keyboard so that it produced a different sound, or combination of sounds, for each key pressed. The sounds would not have to be speech sounds; tones, buzzes, etc., could be used. The sequence of sounds could be tape recorded, and blind people could listen to the tapes or records made from the tapes. A number of different systems were developed. They all were useless, although various schemes for slowing down the tapes, editing them, etc., were tried. Listeners had to slow down the tapes to rates that were about one tenth the rate of normal speech. The blind "readers" would forget what a sentence was about before they heard its end. It made no difference what sort of sounds were connected to the typewriter keys; they were all equally bad. The basic rate of transmission and the inherent difficulty of these systems was about the same as the traditional "dots" and "dashes" of the telegrapher's Morse code, which is very difficult to follow and demands all of your attention.

The solution to this problem seemed to rest in producing speechlike signals. The obvious approach was to make machines that would "glue" the phonetic elements of speech together to make words and sentences. Linguists have traditionally thought of phonetic segments as "beads on a string." There seemed to be no inherent problem if the beads were isolated, collected, and then appropriately strung together. The medium of tape recording seemed to be the solution. Speakers could be recorded while they carefully pronounced words in which the full range of phonetic elements would occur. The phonetic elements could then be isolated by cutting up the magnetic tape (preferably with electronic segmenting devices that were functional equivalents of very precisely controlled scissors). A speaker, for example, would record a list of words that included *pet*, *bat*, *cat*, *hat*, and so on. The experimenters would then theoretically be able to "isolate" the sounds [p], [b], [k], [h], [ɛ], [æ], [t]. The isolated sounds would be stored in a machine that could put them together in different patterns to form new words, for example, *bet* and *pat*. Systems of this sort were attempted (Peterson, Wang and Sivertson 1958), but they did not work. It was, in fact, impossible to isolate individual sounds.

Studies with Vocoder speech synthesizers demonstrated why it was impossible to isolate sounds like the stop consonants [b], [d], and [g]. Figure 7.3 shows a series of synthetic spectrograms that yield the voiced stops [b], [d], and [g] in initial position with various vowels in CV (consonant–vowel) syllables when they are converted to sound on a speech synthesizer (Delattre, Liberman

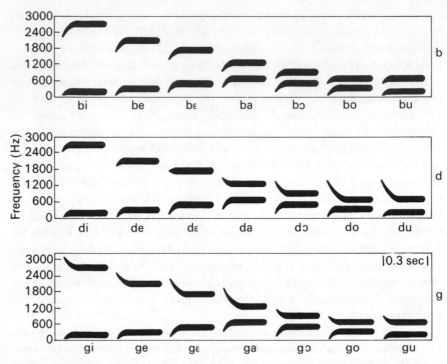

Figure 7.3. Synthetic spectrograms using only F_1 *and* F_2 *information that produce the voiced stops before various vowels. (After Delattre, Liberman and Cooper, 1955.)*

and Cooper, 1955). The synthesizer was controlled with only two formant frequencies and a fundamental frequency control which was uniform for all the stimuli and is not shown in Figure 7.3. The acoustic cues that caused the listeners who identified these stimuli to "hear" the consonants [b], [d], and [g] were the formant transitions, i.e. the changing formant pattern that occurred at the start of each syllable. Note that the formant transitions of the "same" consonant are different for different vowels. It would be impossible to piece together the formant transitions of the [d] of [de] with the vowel [u] to get the syllable [du]. The data of Figure 7.3 show that there are no acoustic segments in these signals that correspond in any way to segmentable "beads." The acoustic realization of a [d] in one syllable is quite different from that in another syllable. Human speech is thus fundamentally different from alphabetic orthography; it is not segmented at the acoustic level. This inherent lack of segmentation is, however, not a liability. It is one of the advantages of human speech as a means of vocal communication. The rate at which meaningful sound distinctions are transmitted in human speech is about 20 to 30 segments per second. That is, phonetic distinctions that differentiate meaningful words,

144

e.g. the sounds symbolized by the notation [b], [æ] and [t] in the word *bat*, are transmitted, identified, and put together at a rate of 20 to 30 segments per second. It is obvious that human listeners cannot simply transmit and identify these sound distinctions as separate entities. The fastest rate at which sounds can be identified is about 7 to 9 segments per second (Miller, 1956). Sounds transmitted at a rate of 20 segments per second merge into an undifferentiable "tone." How, then, is speech transmitted and perceived?

Speech encoding

The results of recent decades of research on the perception of speech by humans demonstrate that the individual sounds like [b], [æ] and [t] are *encoded*, that is "squashed together," into the syllable-sized unit [bæt] (Liberman *et al.*, 1967). A human speaker in producing this syllable starts with his supralaryngeal vocal tract in the shape characteristic of [b]. However, he does not maintain this articulatory configuration, but instead moves his tongue, lips, etc., towards the positions that would be attained if he were instructed to produce an isolated, sustained [æ]. He never reaches these positions because he starts towards the articulatory configuration characteristic of [t] before he reaches the "steady state" (isolated and sustained) [æ] vowel. The articulatory gestures that would be characteristic of each isolated sound are never attained. Instead the articulatory gestures are melded together into a composite, characteristic of the syllable. The sound pattern that results from this encoding process is itself an indivisible composite. There is no way of separating with absolute certainty the [b] articulatory gestures from the [æ] gestures.

The traditional concept of "coarticulation" which derives from classical experimental studies (Rousselot, 1901) cannot, in an absolute sense, account for the encoding of speech. It is possible to locate and isolate segments of the acoustic signal and articulatory gestures that can be closely related to a particular segment, e.g. the vowel [æ] in [bæt]. Speech, however, really does not appear to be perceived, produced, or neurally "programmed" on a segmental basis. Research has yet to reveal invariant motor commands that correspond to the segments of speech (Harris, 1974). If the syllable [bæt] were recorded on a magnetic tape, it would be impossible to isolate either the [b] or the [t]. You would always hear the [æ] vowel. The acoustic cues that, in fact, transmit the initial and final consonants are the modulations of the formant frequency pattern of the [æ] vowel. The process is, in effect, a time-compressing system. The production of the vowel [æ] in the context of an initial and final consonant would always be shorter than that produced in isolation. The effects are pervasive; listeners can recognize the vowel that follows a fricative from the

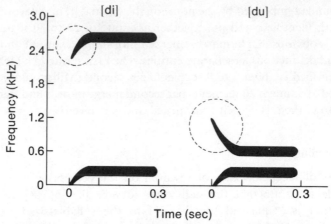

Figure 7.4. Two formant patterns that will produce the sounds [di] and [du]. Note that the second formant frequency transitions are quite different. (After Liberman, 1970a.)

spectral information that is present in the "coarticulated" fricative, e.g. they can identify the [u] of the syllable [su] from the acoustic information transmitted in the [s] (Soli, 1981; Yeni-Komshian and Soli, 1981).

In Figure 7.4 we have reproduced two simplified spectrographic patterns that will, when converted to sound, produce approximations to syllables [di] and [du] (Liberman, 1970a).[1] The dark bands on these patterns represent the first and second formant frequencies as functions of time. Note that the formants rapidly move through a range of frequencies at the left of each pattern. These rapid movements, which occur in about 50 milliseconds, are called *formant transitions*. The transition in the second formant, which is encircled, conveys the minimal acoustic information that human listeners interpret as a token of a [d] in the syllables [di] and [du]. It is again impossible to isolate the acoustic pattern of [d] in these syllables. If tape recordings of these two syllables are "sliced" with the electronic equivalent of a pair of scissors (Liberman, 1970a), it is impossible to find a segment that contains only [d]. There is no way to cut the tape so as to obtain a piece that will produce [d] without also producing the next vowel or some reduced approximation to it. Note that the encircled transitions are different for the two syllables. If these transitions are isolated, listeners report that they hear either an upgoing or a falling frequency modulation. In context, with the acoustic correlates of the entire syllable, these transitions cause listeners to hear an "identical sounding"

[1] It is simpler to start with a single consonant–vowel syllable like [di] or [du], but the principles that we will discuss also apply to longer stretches of speech (Ohman, 1966; MacNeilage, 1970; Lubker and Gay 1982).

[d] in both syllables. How does a human listener effect this perceptual response?

The "motor theory" of speech perception

The formant frequency patterns of speech reflect the resonances of the supralaryngeal vocal tract. The formant patterns that define the syllable [di] in Figure 7.4 thus reflect the changing resonant pattern of the supralaryngeal vocal tract as the speaker moves his articulators from the occlusion of the tongue tip against the palate that is involved in the production of [d] to the vocal tract configuration of the [i]. A different acoustic pattern defines the [d] in the syllable [du]. The resonances of the vocal tract are similar as the speaker forms the initial occlusion of the [d] in both syllables by moving his tongue against his palate (Perkell, 1969); however, the resonances of the vocal tract are quite different for the final configurations of the vocal tract for [i] and [u]. The formant patterns that convey the [d] in both syllables are thus quite different since they involve transitions from the same starting point to different end points. Human listeners "hear" an identical initial [d] segment in both of these signals because they, in effect, "decode" the acoustic pattern using prior "knowledge" of the articulatory gestures and the anatomical apparatus that is involved in the production of speech. The listener in this process, which has been termed the "motor theory of speech perception" (Liberman *et al.*, 1967; Liberman and Mattingly, 1985), operates in terms of the acoustic pattern of the entire syllable. The acoustic cues for the individual "phonetic segments" are fused into a syllabic pattern. The high rate of information transfer of human speech is thus due to the transmission of acoustic information in units that are at least syllable-sized. The phonetic elements of each syllable are "encoded" into a single acoustic pattern which is then "decoded" by the listener to yield the phonetic representation.

In the initial formulation of this theory it was assumed that the listener perceived speech by matching the incoming signal against an internally generated signal. The listener hypothetically generated the internal signal by means of the same neural mechanisms that he used to control his vocal tract in the generation of speech. The process of matching an incoming signal against an internally generated reference was termed "analysis by synthesis" (Halle and Stevens, 1959). Motor theory explanations of various aspects of speech were extended to various aspects of speech perception, including the perception of intonation and stress (Lieberman, 1967). Recent formulations of the motor theory of speech perception (Liberman and Mattingly, 1985) claim that invariant relations exist only at the level of articulation. This extreme formulation of the motor theory claims that a one-to-one mapping exists between a linguistic construct and a motor command. However, these claims are not consistent with the data that have been derived over the past fifty years. We will return to these issues in Chapter 8.

The speech "mode" of perception

When they listen to speech, human listeners often appear to behave in what appears to be a "mode" different from the mode for other acoustic signals. Remez *et al.* (1981) in psychoacoustic experiments that make use of sinusoidal approximations to speech signals show that listeners can either hear the same signals as speech, or as nonspeech "science fiction sounds," "buzzes," etc. The distinctions are abrupt; the same signals are either interpreted as speech signals or not. As speech signals, the acoustic energy of a consonantal formant transition, for example, is heard as a [d]; as a nonspeech sound, it is heard as a chirp. The dominant hemisphere of the brain (which is usually the left hemisphere) appears to be more involved in the perception of speech signals than nonspeech signals. The relevant data include studies of the effects of lesions of the brain (Kimura, 1961, 1967; Penfield and Roberts, 1959; Luria, 1961; Geschwind, 1965), which continue in the tradition of Broca's and Wernicke's original observations. Broca (1861) observed that damage to the brain in a particular area of the left hemisphere will result in a loss of speech production ability. Listeners who have suffered various traumas in their left hemispheres also may have difficulty in perceiving human speech (Wernicke, 1874). The nature of the neural mechanisms that are involved in the production and perception of speech is not known, nor is there general agreement on even the general organization of the brain. The functions of the brain may, or may not, be strictly localized (Penfield and Roberts, 1959). We have to wait until we have a better understanding of the brain before we can identify the specific neural mechanisms that are involved in the perception of speech. There is, however, much evidence that some "specialized" neural processing is involved.

When normal human listeners hear speech sounds, greater electrical potentials are recorded by electrodes positioned over their left hemispheres than over their right hemispheres. In contrast, no differences in electrical activity can be noted by the same electrode array when the subjects listen to musical sounds (McAdam and Whitaker, 1971; Wood, Goff and Day, 1971). The results of hundreds of experiments with dichotically presented speech and nonspeech stimuli (Shankweiler and Studdert-Kennedy, 1967; cf. Bradshaw and Nettleton, 1981; and Bryden, 1982, for reviews) again demonstrate that the left hemisphere of the brain is somehow crucially involved in the perception of speech. The dichotic experiments involve the simultaneous presentation of two different sounds to a listener. One sound is presented to the subject's right ear through one headphone channel. The other, "competing" sound is presented to the subject's left ear via a second headphone channel. Under these conditions, consonant–vowel syllables presented to the subject's right ear tend to be heard more accurately than those presented to the subject's left ear. The effect is manifested statistically; that is, subjects perceive the sound presented to their right ear better than to their left ear.

The effect is most pronounced when speech signals are presented to listeners, but it also occurs for other complex signals (Cutting, 1974; Molfese, 1972). Its basis seems to be the fact that the right ear is connected to the dominant left hemisphere of the brain by a major contralateral pathway.[2] This results in speech and other complex signals that are presented to the right ear "going" more readily to the left hemisphere. The ipsilateral[3] connections of both ears, which transmit signals from the left ear to the left hemisphere and from the right ear to the right hemisphere, prevent the effect from being total. The precise role of the dominant hemisphere in the perception of speech is still not clear; however, it is clear that damage to the left hemisphere has a significant effect on speech perception, whereas damage to the right hemisphere has a minimal effect.

Neural acoustic property detectors

A number of researchers have begun to develop and test models of speech perception that involve neural "property detectors" that respond to specific acoustic signals. Cutting (1974), for example, found that frequency transitions in nonspeech signals are perceived in a manner similar to the formant transitions of consonant–vowel syllables. Human listeners from the age of two months onwards (Eimas *et al.*, 1971; Cutting and Eimas, 1975; Morse, 1972; Molfese, 1972) appear to perceive speech signals in a manner that suggests that the human brain has a number of devices, or property detectors, that respond selectively to particular types of acoustic signals (Cutting and Eimas, 1975). The plausibility of the original motor theory of speech perception comes from the fact that many of these neural property detectors respond to signals that the human vocal tract is adapted to make. In other words, there seems to be a "match" between the sounds that humans can make and the sounds that they are specially adapted to readily perceive (Lieberman, 1970, 1973, 1975, 1984; Stevens, 1972b). People do not have to model internally the maneuvers of the

---

[2] The contralateral pathways are the links that transmit the electrical signal from the right inner ear to the left hemisphere of the brain and the left inner ear to the right hemisphere. The mechanisms of the ear convert acoustic signals into electrical signals (Flanagan, 1972).

[3] The ipsilateral pathways link the right ear to the right hemisphere and the left ear to the left hemisphere. The ipsilateral connections also appear to be effective in transmitting the electrical signals from the inner ear to the brain.

vocal tract and compute the acoustic consequences of possible articulatory patterns in order to determine whether they are listening to a speech sound. They seem to be furnished from birth with neural mechanisms that selectively respond to the acoustic signals of human speech.

Electrophysiological and comparative studies

Studies with animals other than *Homo sapiens* have demonstrated that similar mechanisms exist in their brains. Electrophysiological techniques that cannot be used in experiments with humans have isolated neural mechanisms that respond to signals that are of interest to the animals. These signals include the vocal calls of the animals in question. Even simple animals like crickets appear to have neural units that code information about the rhythmic elements of their mating songs (Hoy and Paul, 1973). Similar results have been obtained in the squirrel monkey (*Saimiri sciureus*). Wollberg and Newman (1972) recorded the electrical activity of single cells in the auditory cortex of awake monkeys during the presentation of recorded monkey vocalizations and other acoustic signals. The electrophysiological techniques of this experiment involved placing electrodes that could record the electrical discharges from 213 cells in the brains of different animals. Some cells responded to many of the calls that had complex acoustic properties. Other cells, however, responded to only a few calls. One cell responded with a high probability only to one specific signal, the "isolation peep" call of the monkey.

The experimental techniques that are necessary in these electrophysiological studies demand great care and great patience. Microelectrodes that can isolate the electrical signal from a single neuron must be prepared and accurately positioned. The electrical signals must be amplified and recorded. Most importantly, the experimenters must present the animals with a set of acoustic signals that explore the range of sounds they would encounter in their natural state. Demonstrating the presence of "neural mechanisms" matched to the constraints of the sound-producing systems of particular animals is therefore a difficult undertaking. The sound-producing possibilities and behavioral responses of most "higher" animals make comprehensive statements on the relationship between perception and production difficult. We can explore only part of the total system of signaling and behavior. However, "simpler" animals are useful in this respect because we can see the whole pattern of their behavior.

The behavioral experiments of Capranica (1965) and the electrophysiological experiments of Frishkopf and Goldstein (1963), for example, demonstrate that the auditory system of the bullfrog (*Rana catesbiana*) has single units that are matched to the formant frequencies of the species-specific mating call. Bullfrogs are members of the class Amphibia. Frogs and toads compose the order Anura. They are the simplest living animals that produce sound by means of a laryngeal source and a supralaryngeal vocal tract (Stuart, 1958). The supralaryngeal vocal tract consists of a mouth, a pharynx, and a vocal sac that opens into the floor of the mouth in the male. Vocalizations are produced in the same manner as in primates; the vocal folds of the larynx open and close rapidly, emitting "puffs" of air into the supralaryngeal vocal tract, which acts as an acoustic filter. Frogs can make a number of different calls (Bogert, 1960), including mating calls, release calls, territorial calls that serve as warnings to intruding frogs, rain calls, distress calls, and warning calls. The different calls have distinct acoustic properties, and there are obvious differences in the manner in which frogs produce some calls. For example, the distress call is made with the frog's mouth wide open, whereas all other calls are made with the mouth closed. The articulatory distinctions that underlie the other calls are not as obvious. Capranica (1965) has, however, analyzed the acoustic properties of the bullfrog mating call in detail.

The mating call of the bullfrog consists of a series of croaks. The duration of a croak varies from 0.6 to 1.5 seconds and the interval between croaks from 0.5 to 1.0 second. The fundamental frequency of the bullfrog croak is about 0.1 kHz. The formant frequencies of the croak are about 0.2 and 1.4 kHz. Capranica generated synthetic frog croaks by means of a POVO speech synthesizer (Stevens, Bastide and Smith, 1955), a fixed speech synthesizer designed to produce human vowels that serves equally well for the synthesis of bullfrog croaks. In a behavioral experiment, Capranica showed that bullfrogs responded to synthesized croaks so long as there were energy concentrations at either or both of the formant frequencies that characterize the natural croak. The presence of acoustic energy at other frequencies inhibited the bullfrogs' responses. (The bullfrogs' responses consisted of joining in a croak chorus.)

Frishkopf and Goldstein (1963), in their electrophysiological study of the bullfrog's auditory system, found two types of auditory units. They found cells in units in the eighth cranial nerve of the anesthetized bullfrog that had maximum sensitivity to frequencies between 1.0 and 2.0 kHz and other units that had maximum sensitivity to frequencies between 0.2 and 0.7 kHz. However, the units that responded to the lower frequency range were inhibited by appropriate acoustic signals. Maximum response occurred when the two units responded to time-locked pulse trains at rates of 50 and 100 pulses per second that had energy concentrations at, or near, the formant frequencies of bullfrog mating calls. Adding acoustic energy between the two formant frequencies at 0.5 kHz inhibited the responses of the low frequency single units.

The electrophysiological, behavioral, and acoustic data all complement each other. Bullfrogs have auditory mechanisms that are structured to respond specifically to the bullfrog mating call. Bullfrogs do not respond to just any sort of acoustic signal as though it were a mating call; they respond to particular calls that have the acoustic properties of those that can be made only by male bullfrogs, and they have neural mechanisms structured in terms of the species-specific constraints of the bullfrog sound-producing mechanism. Capranica tested his bullfrogs with the mating calls of 34 other species of frog, and they responded only to bullfrog calls, ignoring all others. The croaks have to have energy concentrations equivalent to those that would be produced by both formant frequencies of the bullfrogs' supralaryngeal vocal tract. Furthermore, the stimuli have to have the appropriate fundamental frequency.

The bullfrog has one of the simplest forms of sound-making systems that can be characterized by the source–filter theory of sound production. Its perceptual apparatus is demonstrably structured in terms of the constraints of its sound-producing apparatus and the acoustic parameters of the source–filter theory – the fundamental frequency and formant frequencies. The neural property detectors that appear to be involved in the perception of human speech are more complex in so far as human speech involves a greater variety of sounds. The acoustic properties of vowels and of sounds like the stop consonants [b], [p], [d], [t], etc., are, for example, quite different. The discrimination and identification of these different classes of sounds also differ and may reflect the presence of different types of neural acoustic property detectors.

Psychoacoustic tests

Discrimination versus identification of sounds

Much of the perceptual data that we have cited in connection with the probable existence of neural acoustic property detectors in humans involves the phenomenon of "categorical discrimination." In order to understand the significance of categorical discrimination and indeed to understand the terminology we first must clearly understand the distinction that exists between the *discrimination* and the *identification* of speech sounds and other stimuli. These two terms signify very different perceptual tasks. The examples that follow may perhaps make the distinction clear. Suppose that you have a friend who wishes to test your ability to discriminate between the sounds that the different keys of a piano produce when they are struck. Your friend seats you with your back to the piano and strikes a particular key. He then produces another sound on his piano. You do not know whether he has hit the same key again, or has instead hit a different key. He asks you to tell him whether the second sound is like the first sound or whether it is different. If he sometimes randomly hits the same key twice you cannot automatically say that the two sounds are always different. You will have to listen carefully to each pair of sounds that he produces. If the experiment were run using careful controls, e.g. striking the different keys with equal force, your friend would be able to determine your ability to discriminate between the sounds that the different keys of the piano produce. The chances are that you would be able to discriminate between all of the keys of the piano if you had normal hearing and if the piano were in good repair and tune.

The results of an identification test would probably be quite different. Suppose that your friend wanted to test your ability to identify the sounds that the keys of his piano produced. You again might start with your back to the piano. Your friend would strike the keys of the piano in a random order and ask you to identify the note that was produced by each key. He would not strike the keys in an ascending or descending scale. Even if you had musical training you would find the task difficult unless you are one of the rare individuals who has perfect pitch. Psychoacoustic tests with pure sinusoidal tones show that most people can reliably identify no more than about four or five different tones (Pollack, 1952). If you had normal hearing and could hear the frequency range between 20 and 20 000 Hz, you could, in contrast, discriminate between about 350 000 different sinusoidal tones (S. S. Stevens and Davis, 1938). Psychoacoustic experiments have established the difference limens (dl's) for the minimal differences that humans can perceive in fundamental frequency, formant frequencies, vowel amplitude (Flanagan, 1955a, 1955b), timing (Hirsch, 1959), etc. The difference between discrimination and identification is similar for other sensory tasks. It is, for example, easy to discriminate between colors but it is hard to make absolute identifications. Consider the problems that you may have when you try to identify the color of a particular shade of paint in a store (to match it with the color of some object at home) and the subsequent ease with which you and others can discriminate between the two slightly different paint colors once you have patched a scratch with the new batch of paint. Discrimination is an easier task than identification; you can readily discriminate between a set of objects that you cannot reliably identify.

Psychoacoustic tests are a necessary part of speech research. Although it is possible to perform precise analyses of speech signals using electronic instruments and computer programs that effect various mathematical transformations of the signal, these analyses are, in themselves, meaningless. We can never be certain that we have actually isolated the acoustic cues that people use to transmit information to each other unless we run psychoacoustic studies in which human listeners respond to acoustic signals that differ with respect to the acoustic cues that we think are relevant. Speech synthesizers are thus very useful tools since they permit us to generate acoustic signals that differ with respect to some particular attribute. It is foolish to assume that you can isolate a linguistically relevant acoustic cue without running psychoacoustic experiments, even when the acoustic cue seems to be very "simple." Bloomfield (1933, p. 110), for example, assumed that the acoustic factor that determined the perceptual "loudness" of a sound was the physical intensity of the speech signal. He was wrong. Humans are not electronic instruments that directly respond to a physical measure like intensity. Human judgements of loudness turn out to be a function of the duration and amplitude of the sound (Lifschitz, 1933). Bloomfield further supposed that the relative loudness of the syllables of words like *rébel* and *rebél* was the basis of the contrast in linguistic "stress" that differentiates these word pairs. The word that bears stress on the first syllable (which is indicated by the symbol ´) is the noun form, e.g. *The rébel stood in the doorway*. The verb form bears stress on its second syllable, e.g. *You must rebél from your sorry state*. Many verb and noun forms in English are differentiated, in part, by stress.

Psychoacoustic tests (Fry, 1955; Lieberman, 1965) and acoustic analyses (Lieberman, 1960, 1967; Morton and Jassem, 1965; Atkinson, 1973) show that human listeners make seemingly "simple" stress distinctions by taking into account the total fundamental frequency contour of the utterance, the amplitude of syllabic "peaks," the relative durations of segments of the utterance and the range of formant frequency variations. What seems "simple" to us involves a complex decision-making procedure when we try to make stress decisions with an artificial automaton (Lieberman, 1960). The responses of human listeners to even "simple" nonspeech stimuli like sinusoidal signals is not simple. Psychoacoustic "scaling" experiments show that judgements of the relative pitch of two sinusoids are not equivalent to their arithmetic frequency ratio (Beranek, 1949; Fant, 1973; Nearey, 1976, 1978). In other words, if you let a human listener hear a sinusoid whose frequency is 1000 Hz and then let him adjust the control of a frequency generator until he hears a sound that has twice the pitch of the 1000 Hz signal, he will not set the control to 2000 Hz. He will instead select a sinusoid whose frequency is about 3100 Hz. Judgement of relative perceived pitch can be related to the physical measure of frequency by the use of a "Mel" conversion scale. The Mel scale which relates perceived pitch to frequency is plotted in Figure 7.5. Note that the perceptual ratio between two frequencies depends on the absolute magnitude of the frequencies. Frequency is plotted against the horizontal axis in Figure 7.5. The perceptual Mel equivalent of a frequency is plotted with respect to the vertical axis. A sinusoid whose frequency is 1000 Hz thus has a Mel value of 1000 Mel and is twice the pitch of a sinusoid having a pitch of 500 Mel. The frequency of a sinusoid having a pitch of 500 Mel is 400 Hz. A sound whose pitch is 3000 Mel will have twice the perceived pitch of 1500 Mel but the frequency ratio of these two sounds is 9000/2000. The Mel scale is of particular value in regard to some of the acoustic relations that structure the phonetic theory of vowels that we will discuss in Chapter 8.

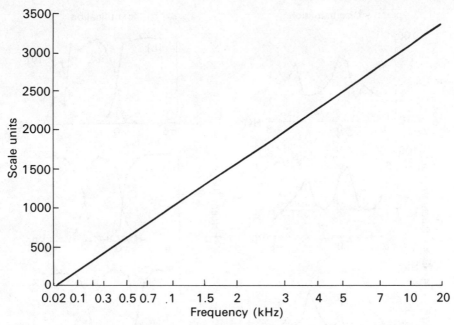

Figure 7.5. The Mel scale which relates perceived pitch to frequency. (Adapted from Fant, 1973.)

Categorical perception

It is straightforward to design psychoacoustic experiments that test either the discrimination or the identification of speech sounds. The speech stimuli can be samples of "real speech," i.e. produced by humans, or "synthetic speech" produced by speech synthesizers that use either terminal or area function analogs of the vocal tract. Whereas certain speech sounds, like vowels, behave like nonspeech stimuli in so far as discrimination is much "better" than identification, the discrimination of other speech sounds is very different. Sounds like the English stop consonants are discriminated no better than they are identified. The graphs of Figure 7.6 illustrate this phenomenon, which has been termed "categorical perception." The graphs in the right-hand column show the results of an identification experiment in which listeners had to identify synthesized speech sounds (Liberman, 1970b). The test stimuli were produced on a terminal analog synthesizer with two formants and a specified fundamental frequency. The formant frequency patterns were like those shown in Figure 7.7. The first formant pattern was the same for all of the stimuli. The starting point of the second formant transition varied. Depending on the starting point of the second formant, the sounds were identified as examples of the syllables [bæ], [dæ], or [gæ]. As Figure 7.7 shows, the formant

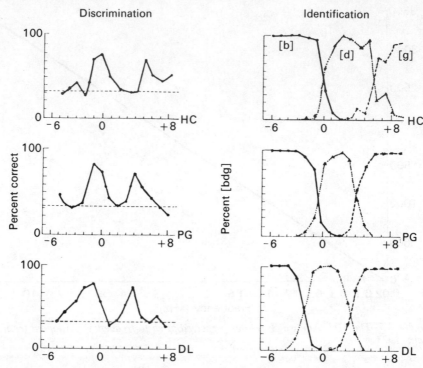

Figure 7.6. Identification and discrimination functions for three different listeners responding to synthetic speech stimuli that are cued by the second formant transitions schematized in Figure 7.7. The three listeners are HC, PG, and DL. The synthesized sounds are heard as [bæ], [dæ], and [gæ]. The numbers on the horizontal scale of the figures refer to the second formant frequency transitions numbered in Figure 7.7. (Adapted from Liberman, 1970b.)

frequencies of F_2 were numbered with reference to whether the formant frequency was the same as the F_2 of the vowel (stimulus 0). Stimuli with F_2 starting frequencies lower than the vowel steady-state were given consecutive negative values. Thus, stimuli -1 to -6 had *rising transitions*. Stimuli with F_2 starting frequencies higher than the vowel steady-state were given consecutive positive values. Thus, stimuli $+1$ to $+9$ had *falling transitions*. Stimulus number -6, the first stimulus on the continuum, had a starting F_2 frequency of about 1100 Hz; stimulus number $+2$, the ninth stimulus on the continuum, had a starting F_2 frequency of about 1800 Hz; and stimulus $+9$, the last stimulus on the continuum, had a starting F_2 frequency of about 2350 Hz. The graphs in the right-hand column in Figure 7.6 show that listener HC labeled, i.e. identified, stimuli -6 to -1 as examples of [bæ] stimuli 0 to 5 as [dæ], and

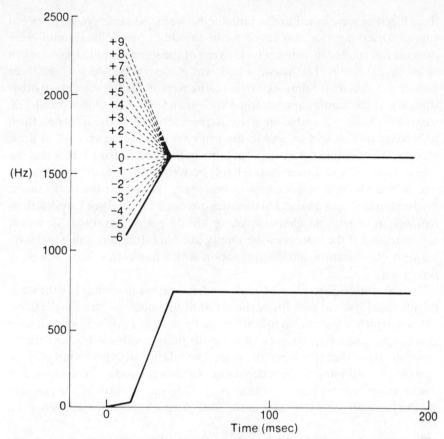

Figure 7.7. Schematic representation of two formant frequency patterns that will produce the sounds [bæ], [dæ], and [gæ]. The numbers – 6 through +9 reference the different signals. (Adapted from Liberman, 1970b).

stimuli 6 to 9 as [gæ], etc. The graph shows, for example, that stimulus –4 was identified 100 percent of the time as [bæ] by all three listeners. Note that subjects' responses change rather abruptly. They identify a series of stimuli as [b], and rather abruptly change their responses to [d] for a number of stimuli, and then again abruptly change their responses to [g]. The boundaries between the identified categories [b], [d] and [g] occur where the identification curves for each category fall and overlap. The category boundary can be computed as that point along the continuum where identification responses are 50 percent. In the case of the [b d g] continuum, there are two category boundaries, one between [b] and [d] and the other between [d] and [g].

The graphs in the left-hand column of Figure 7.6 show what happened when these listeners were asked to discriminate between the same synthetic speech stimuli. Discrimination was tested using an oddity procedure. Stimuli were presented in triads consisting of two tokens of the same stimuli and one token of another stimulus. The listener's task was to determine which of the three stimuli was different. Stimulus comparisons were made between every other stimulus on the continuum, i.e. stimulus -6 and -4, stimulus -5 and -3, stimulus -4 and -2, and so on. If the listeners acted as we should expect them to behave, they should be able to discriminate reliably between all of these stimuli. The graphs in the left-hand column in Figure 7.6 instead show that the listeners were able to discriminate reliably between these sounds *only* when the pair of sounds lie across a category boundary. Note that the peaks in the discrimination function occur at the category boundaries. Elsewhere discrimination is at or near the chance level, i.e. the 33 percent level that we would expect to find if the listeners were simply guessing. It is this unique relation between identification and discrimination which has been called *categorical perception*.

The categorical perception of adult human listeners to sounds like the stops [b], [d], and [g] could perhaps be the result of unconscious "training" (Lane, 1965) in which listeners respond differentially to sound distinctions that have great importance. Experiments with one- to four-month-old human infants, however, show that this is not the case. The infants' discrimination of these stimuli also appears to be categorical. In other words, the infants also discriminate between pairs of stimuli only when one member of the pair is in the [bæ] category and the other in the [dæ] category (cf. Jusczyk, 1986, for a review).

However, it is important to note that the labeling functions which we are describing are those of the adults. The infants are only presented with stimulus pairs to discriminate. It is of course impossible actually to ask the infants to label the test stimuli. Because we cannot directly compare labeling and discrimination functions for infants, we cannot say they show categorical perception. Rather, we can only claim that they show *categorical discrimination* and their perception of speech seems to be *categorical-like* in that their discrimination functions are similar to those obtained for adults. These categorical-like effects disappear when the isolated transitions of the second formant (which are the sole acoustic variables in these experiments) are presented in isolation. These stimuli are no longer perceived by adult listeners as speech, but as "chirps" or glissandos of frequency change. Adult (Mattingly *et al.*, 1971) and infant (Cutting and Eimas, 1975) listeners under these conditions are able to discriminate between all the isolated second formant transitions. Thus, the same acoustic variable (the F_2 formant transition) is perceived categorically only when it is incorporated as part of the speech stimulus. When it is presented in isolation, and no longer heard as speech, the stimuli are not perceived categorically. We will discuss the acquisition of speech by children in more detail in Chapter 9.

Critical bands

The perception of speech is necessarily structured by the inherent constraints of the auditory system. Much recent work has been directed at determining how the auditory system constrains the way in which we process speech sounds (Delgutte, 1980; Goldhor, 1984). Although many aspects of the auditory system are not clearly understood, the concept of "critical bands" has proved productive.

The term *critical band* has been used in several different ways in the literature. Originally, it was used by Fletcher (1940) with respect to the masking of a tone by noise. He wanted to know how much of the noise actually contributed to the masking of a tone. In other words, he asked whether the entire bandwidth of the noise spectrum contributed to masking or whether there is a certain limited bandwidth or "critical bandwidth" of the noise that is responsible for the masking of the tone. He found that indeed only a certain critical band of the noise, a bandwidth that centered around that of the tone, actually masked the tone.

If we consider a critical band as though it were a filter with a certain bandwidth, then the results of such studies as those of Fletcher and others become clear-cut. What they suggest is that the ear or more generally the auditory system serves as a band of filters. Psychophysical and electrophysiological research has attempted to determine what is the nature of this filtering process. Results have shown that the critical band, i.e. that bandwidth at which subjective responses of listeners change abruptly (Sharf, 1970), varies as a function of frequency. Figure 7.8 summarizes these results. Note that at 1000 Hz the critical band is 200 Hz, whereas at 10 000 Hz, the critical band is 1000 Hz. This means that the listener's sensitivity to frequency changes are not the same across the frequency range: At the lower frequencies, the auditory system acts as a narrower filter than it does at higher frequencies. Thus, it is more sensitive to frequency changes at lower than higher frequencies. Table 7.1 provides a summary of the values obtained for auditory critical bands (from Zwicker, 1961). If you plot out the center frequency, bandwidth, and cut-off frequencies, you will note that the critical bands represent a set of overlapping filters rather than discrete, contiguous filters, and that their size and shape vary along the frequency scale. It has been suggested that critical bands represent equal distances (about 1.3 mm) along the basilar membrane of the ear (Greenwood, 1961), although others suggest

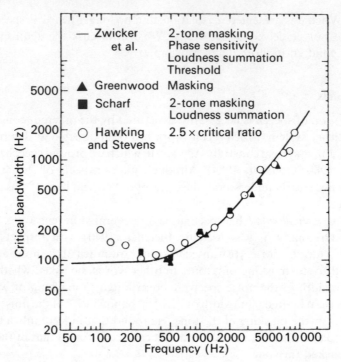

Figure 7.8. Critical bandwidth as a function of the frequency at the center of the band. The solid line is a smoothed average of measurements by Zwicker and his colleagues. Triangles (Greenwood, 1961) are based upon masking by narrow bands of noise. Squares are averages obtained by Sharf (1970). Circles are the published signal-to-noise ratios of Hawking and Stevens (1950) converted to hertz and multiplied by 2.5. (From Zwicker, 1961.)

that critical bands correspond to neural density in the cochlea (Zwislocki, 1965). Whichever results are correct, it is clear that the auditory system filters the acoustic signal in very particular ways, and helps "shape" the perception of the auditory properties of speech.

Exercises

1. Strict adherents of the motor theory of speech perception claim that there is an invariant relationship between articulation and the linguistic distinctions that are conveyed in speech. Do you agree with this, and why?

2. Why are auditory constraints like "critical bands" significant factors in the perception of speech?

3. Explain "categorical perception."

Table 7.1. *Critical bands (from Zwicker, 1961)*

Number	Center frequencies (Hz)	Cut-off frequencies (Hz)	Bandwidth (Hz)
1	50	100	80
2	150	200	100
3	250	300	100
4	350	400	100
5	450	510	110
6	570	630	120
7	700	770	140
8	840	920	150
9	1000	1080	160
10	1170	1270	190
11	1370	1480	210
12	1600	1720	240
13	1850	2000	280
14	2150	2320	320
15	2500	2700	380
16	2900	3150	450
17	3400	3700	550
18	4000	4400	700
19	4800	5300	900
20	5800	6400	1100
21	7000	7700	1300
22	8500	9500	1800
23	10 500	12 000	2500
24	13 500	15 500	3500

8

Phonetic theories

Phonetic theories, like all scientific theories, depend on a particular database and the research techniques that are used to derive that database. Phonetic theories relate the physical attributes of sounds with their linguistic function. Thus the linguistic relevance of particular sounds must be considered as well as acoustical and articulatory data. We could provide an "exact" recording of the speech sounds of a language by making a set of tape recordings which would preserve all of the acoustic attributes of the signals that served as a medium of vocal communication. However, we would not have isolated the linguistically significant phonetic elements that were used in this language. We would not, for example, be able to predict the possible words of this language. We could start on a phonetic analysis of these tape recordings by listening to them and attempting to isolate phonetic elements. Of course, we would be abstracting elements from the encoded stream of sounds using our internal speech-decoding devices. Our task would be simpler if we had also recorded native speakers producing isolated words, and it would be much simpler if we had the services of a bilingual "informant" who spoke our language and the language that we were attempting to analyze.

It would be best if we were analyzing our own native language, but we would nonetheless have to remember that we could not derive the acoustic correlates of phonetic elements without making use of acoustic analysis, synthesis, and psychoacoustic experiments. We would know that the encoded nature of speech meant that we could not easily expect to find separable acoustic segments that would directly correlate with phonetic elements. We would know, however that it is possible to represent speech in terms of a sequence of discrete symbols. All alphabetic, orthographic systems make use of a phonetic or quasi-phonetic system. The relationship between a symbol and a sound is sometimes more variable, i.e. more subject to various rules or odd variations, in some languages than in other languages. All alphabetic systems, however, depend on the fact that it is possible to represent sounds by discrete symbols. Our traditional alphabetic orthography lets us generate sound sequences that convey information, but it does not explain how we are able to produce recognizable sounds when we see these transcriptions.

The ends of a scientific phonetic theory are to "explain" how we produce meaningful sounds, how these sounds may be structured in terms of linguistically relevant units and how they reflect the biology of the human speech/language system. The only way that we can test a scientific theory is to see what data it "explains." Scientific theories, if they are useful, relate things that previously were thought to be unrelated. Newton thus related the motions of the planets and the motion of objects on Earth when he demonstrated that the same mathematical "rules" would predict the motion of planets and cannon balls. Phonetic theories that predict the possible range of sounds of human languages, the relative frequency of occurrence of various sounds, the sequence of events in the acquisition of speech by infants, the most likely types of sound changes, or the effects of various craniofacial anomalies on speech are thus "better" theories than ones that do not make these predictions. Phonetic theories must be able to provide an explanatory basis for real physical data, and they may lead to practical and useful applications.

Traditional "articulatory" phonetic theory

The traditional phonetic theory that is most familiar to speech scientists and linguists was developed during the nineteenth century. Melville Bell (1867) did most to develop this theory although he probably derived it from earlier works (Nearey, 1978). Bell was concerned with finding a set of articulatory maneuvers that he could teach to deaf people that would enable them to talk. The focus of his system therefore was to find articulatory maneuvers that would serve as "instructions" for producing various sounds. Many of the articulatory maneuvers that are involved in speech production are evident. The position of the lips in sounds like the vowel [u] (the vowel of *boot*), for example, can be observed without any special instruments and was noted in many earlier phonetic theories. Some articulatory maneuvers that cannot be directly observed had also been incorporated in earlier phonetic theories, e.g. the maneuvers of the larynx that produce voicing. The physiological research of the late eighteenth and early nineteenth century had determined the role of the larynx in producing and regulating phonation. Bell also used several hypothetical articulatory features that specified the position of a presumed "point of constriction" formed by the tongue against the palate in the oral cavity.

The articulatory theory that derives from Bell's studies has become the "classic" phonetic theory. It has provided the key for significant advances in phonetics, phonology, and speech pathology. The hypotheses that Bell and his successors proposed have been extremely productive; recent research, however, indicates that certain aspects of this theory have to be modified. Although

163

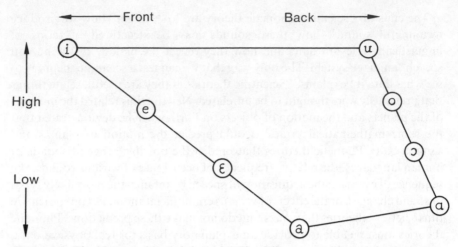

Figure 8.1. The IPA vowel "quadrilateral." The different vowels are defined in terms of the hypothetical position of the tongue. The articulatory dimensions are front versus back, and high versus low.

the theory appears to be in accord with articulatory data for consonants, it fails to account for many aspects of vowel production.

Vowels

Bell believed that the phonetic quality of vowels derived from the position and height of the point of constriction of the tongue. The height of the tongue constriction was supposed to be low for a vowel like [a], whereas it was supposed to be high for vowels like [i] and [u]. The position of the point of constriction with respect to the front-to-back dimension of the oral cavity was also specified. The point of constriction was front for [i] and back for [u]. Bell's original articulatory notation was abandoned, but his theory was preserved with comparatively few modifications. A typical vowel diagram that specifies the vowels of English is shown in Figure 8.1. The overall shape of the presumed vowel space differs somewhat in different versions of this articulatory classification scheme. The "low" vowels sometimes form a quadrilateral space, sometimes a triangle, but the basic dimensions of front–back and high–low are preserved. Individual vowels like [e] (the vowel of *bait*) can be specified in terms of relative position to other vowels. The vowel [e] can thus be described as a front, high vowel somewhat lower than [i] but higher than [ɛ] (the vowel of *bet*). It is also possible to assign numbers to the degrees of height, so [e] could be classified as having height 4 on a scale of 1 to 5, where [i] has 5, the highest value. Bell's theory is essentially preserved in the "generative" theory of Chomsky and Halle (1968) where a number of binary features specify the height and position of the tongue. The use of binary notation in itself does not mean that binary values are being assigned to an articulatory parameter. (A binary number system can be used to represent numbers that can also be expressed in terms of other number bases.)

Bell's articulatory features specifying tongue position were made without the benefit of radiographic data. Bell was therefore unaware of the role of the pharyngeal cavity in the production of speech. He was concerned with the position of the presumed "point of constriction" in the oral cavity. Various techniques were employed to obtain data that would test and refine this theory. Direct palatography, for example, involved coating the palate with a substance that would wipe off when the tongue came in contact with the palate. A subject would produce a sound after having his palate coated and then open his mouth for inspection. Indirect palatography involved placing a metal form, that generally conformed to the contours of the palate, in the subject's mouth while he produced a sound. The surface of the metal form that would come into contact with the tongue could be coated with lampblack or some other substance that would smudge when it came into contact with the tongue. The metal form could be examined after the speaker had produced the appropriate sound, to see where along the palate the constriction was made.

Testing the traditional vowel theory

It is relatively simple to test the components of a phonetic theory that describes vowel production in terms of articulatory gestures if X-rays are available. It is possible to produce sustained vowels so that the problems of encoding sequences of sounds can be avoided. Radiographic techniques made X-rays of the supralaryngeal vocal tract possible by 1919 (Jones, 1919). Russell (1928) made use of radiographs of sustained vowels spoken by speakers of American English. His radiographic data are not as refined as the data of recent studies, but he correctly noted that the data were not consistent with Melville Bell's hypotheses concerning tongue height and the front–back distinction of vowels. Recent cineradiographic studies that allow the analysis of speech under more natural conditions demonstrate that Russell was correct.

Figure 8.2 is reproduced from a study of Ladefoged and his associates (Ladefoged *et al.*, 1972). Note that the tongue contour is almost identical for the vowels [ɪ], [ɛ], and [e]. The tongue is higher for the vowel [i], but differences in tongue contour *cannot* be the factors that differentiate the vowels [ɪ], [ɛ], and [e]. In Figure 8.3, data for a second speaker are presented. Note that there are differences in tongue contour for all of these "front" vowels. However, contrary to traditional vowel theory, the tongue contour for the vowel [e] is

165

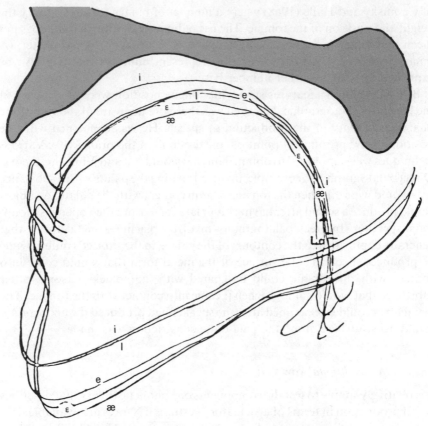

Figure 8.2. Radiographic data derived from an X-ray movie of a speaker producing various English vowels. The tongue contours were sketched from motion picture frames that were exposed during the most stable part of each vowel's articulation. Note the lack of differentiation for the different vowels. The contour of the mandible is also sketched. (After Ladefoged et al., *1972.)*

"higher" than the vowel [ɪ]. In Figure 8.4 we finally see evidence from a speaker whose vowels are produced in accord with traditional vowel theory. It is clear, however, that different speakers behave differently, and, except for the vowel [i], which has a consistent contour in these data (Ladefoged *et al.*, 1972) and in the data of Perkell (1969) and Nearey (1978), the acoustic differences that differentiate these vowels must be the result of the total supralaryngeal vocal tract area function. The speakers make small adjustments in the size of their lip opening, the relative protrusion or retraction of their lips, and the height of their larynges.

The formant frequency patterns that specify particular vowels are deter-

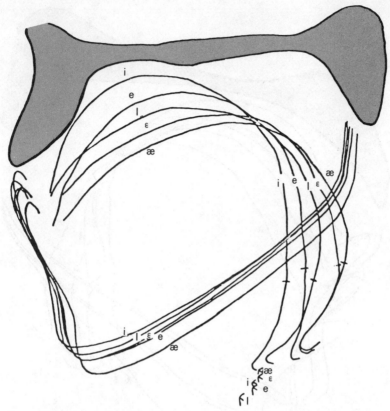

Figure 8.3. Radiographic data for a second speaker. There is more differentiation with respect to the tongue contours, but note that the vowel [e] is "higher" than the vowel [ɪ]. (After Ladefoged et al., 1972.)

mined by the shape and size of the total supralaryngeal airway (Fant, 1960); in other words, the cross-sectional area, as a function of distance from the larynx, of the air passages. The traditional articulatory dimensions of tongue "height" and "frontness" or "backness" would be meaningful if these parameters were significant with regard to specifying the total supralaryngeal vocal tract area functions of different sounds. The data (Nearey, 1978; Ladefoged *et al.*, 1972; Russell, 1928), however, show that the tongue contour, in itself, is not an invariant specification of the supralaryngeal vocal tract area functions that generate the acoustic signals of these different vowels. Nearey (1978), using cineradiographic data derived from three adult speakers of American English, shows that neither the total shape of the tongue contour nor the position of the point of maximum constriction of the tongue against the palate correlate with the claims of traditional articulatory phonetic theories. Except for vowels like

167

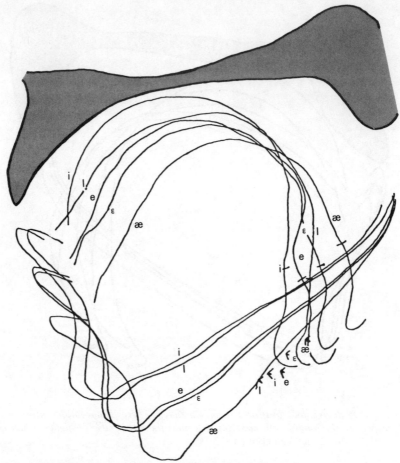

Figure 8.4. Radiographic data for a third speaker, whose tongue contours are in accord with the traditional articulatory classification. All three of these speakers (cf. Figures 8.2, 8.3, and 8.4), however, produced appropriate acoustic signals for all of these vowels although they used different articulatory maneuvers. (After Ladefoged et al., 1972.)

[i], [u] and [a], a "low" back vowel does not necessarily have a lower tongue position than a "high" vowel produced by the same speaker. Similar conclusions follow from the cineradiographic data of Perkell (1969) that we mentioned in Chapter 6. As Perkell noted, differences in larynx height and lip protrusion and constriction are responsible for the formant frequency distinctions that specify vowels like [ɪ], [ɛ] and [e] for the speaker whose utterances he analyzed. Differences in tongue contour can generate appropriate area functions (Figure 8.4), but that is only one possibility.

168

These data are in accord with the predictions of the modeling study of Stevens and House (1955) which we discussed in Chapter 6. The study demonstrated that most vowels can be generated by means of many different articulatory patterns. The only vowels that needed particular tongue contours were ones like [i], [u], and [a], which involved extreme departures from the "neutral" position of the vocal tract. All other vowels can be generated by adjustments of lip opening and total vocal tract length. The human larynx has a vertical mobility of almost 20 mm (Perkell, 1969) so the total range of vocal tract length adjustment is quite great when the effects of lip protrusion and lip retraction are added in. The effects of lip opening are functionally equivalent to adjustments of overall vocal tract length (Stevens and House, 1955). Human speakers, thus, in general do not generate vowels in accordance with traditional phonetic theory.

It is important to note that a human listener cannot tell whether a speaker produced a vowel like [e] by maneuvering his tongue (like the speaker of Figure 8.4) or by maneuvering his lips and larynx (like the speakers of Figure 8.2 and 8.3) unless the "listener" is equipped with X-ray vision or insists on holding conversations in front of X-ray machines. Inferences that follow from the auditory impression of a "trained phonetician" must be regarded as initial hypotheses. The situation is not very different for samples of speech from speakers of four African languages (Asante Twi, Igbo, Dho-Luo, and Ateso) and German discussed by Lindau, Jacobson and Ladefoged (1972). While the tongue shapes that differentiate particular vowel contrasts of some of these speakers seem to be more directly related to a muscular maneuver that shifts the tongue root forward, in some cases the speakers produced similar acoustic contrasts by means of other gestures. As Lindau, Jacobson and Ladefoged (1972) noted,

> The nature of some vowel targets is much more likely to be auditory than articulatory. The particular articulatory mechanism that a speaker makes use of to attain a vowel target is of secondary importance only (p.93).

In summary, the deficiencies of traditional articulation-based phonetic theory involve two related points. First, formant frequency patterns that differentiate many speech sounds are determined by the area function of the supralaryngeal vocal tract. A particular area function will always result in a specified, unique formant frequency pattern. This would seem to support the traditional specification of sounds in terms of invariant articulatory patterns. However, for many vowels, different area functions can produce the same formant frequency patterns. The computer modeling studies of Stevens and House (1955) showed that this was a theoretical possibility. Second, the X-ray studies that we have reviewed, together with many other studies, demonstrate that normal adult speakers actually make use of different articulatory maneuvers to effect similar phonetic contrasts. Although some speakers make use of articulatory maneuvers that afford a reasonable fit with the traditional articulatory parameters (tongue height and the front–back distinction), other speakers produce equivalent acoustic signals by means of very different articulatory maneuvers.

A physiological theory for vowels

The deficiencies of traditional vowel theory arise from the fact that phonetic contrasts are directly related to invariant articulatory maneuvers. These particular deficiencies can be avoided by a "unified" theory that is structured in terms of both articulatory and perceptual factors (Ladefoged *et al.*, 1972; Lieberman, 1970, 1976; Lindau, Jacobson and Ladefoged, 1972; Nearey, 1978). In other words, the phonetic theory is structured in terms of the biological mechanisms that are involved in the production and the perception of speech. Like most theories, this theory follows from "old" theories and it owes much to the theory proposed in *Preliminaries to speech analysis* (Jakobson, Fant and Halle, 1963). Jakobson and his colleagues proposed that the sounds of speech could be specified in terms of a set of "distinctive features," each of which had well-defined acoustic "correlates." The distinctive features, although they were related to articulatory maneuvers that could produce the desired acoustic correlate, focused on the acoustic and linguistic aspects of the sounds of speech. Since the time of the Sanskrit and Greek grammarians of the fourth and fifth centuries BC, linguists have noted that the sounds of speech are often modified in what appear to be regular patterns. Thus, in English, the final sound of the plural form of a "regular" noun that ends with a stop consonant depends on whether the final stop is, or is not, voiced. Compare, for example, the plural forms of the words *light* and *bag*, i.e. *light* + *s* and *bag* + *z*. As we noted in Chapters 6 and 7, the sounds of speech can either be − *voiced* or + *voiced*. Voicing thus appears to be a phonetic feature that specifies a linguistically relevant acoustic property of speech sounds. Jakobson argued for a particular set of universal phonetic features that could only have binary values. The results of many acoustic and psychoacoustic experiments and recent insights on the possible nature of neural acoustic property detectors are not in accord with the detailed acoustic correlates of many of these initial hypothetical features, nor do they support the view that all phonetic features are necessarily binary (cf. Ladefoged, 1975). However, these data are consistent with the central focus of Jakobson's theory − the focus on acoustic factors that are, in turn, based on the constraints of speech production.

The biological or physiological approach that we shall develop in this discussion of a phonetic theory for vowels will attempt to "explain" some of the observed properties of vowel sounds. Physiology is the study of biological function. The physiological approach that we will follow was first proposed by Johannes Müller, who was one of the founders of both modern physiology and psychology. Müller observed (1848) that some of the sounds of human speech appeared to be more basic than others. Purkinje's linguistic studies (1836), for example, showed that certain sounds, like the vowels [i] and [u], appeared to occur more often in different languages. Müller wondered whether these differences reflected the physiological value of particular sounds, and he stated that the *explanations* for these functional differences in the occurrence of these sounds must follow from their physiological attributes. As Müller noted (1848, p.1044), "It comes within the province of physiology to investigate the natural classification of the sounds of language."

Quantal vowels

As we have noted before, the shape of the supralaryngeal vocal tract determines the particular acoustic signal, and different speech sounds are specified by different acoustic signals. Each different sound can involve different maneuvers of the tongue, lips, velum, etc., as the speaker talks. If the speaker could produce vocal tract shapes with maximum precision, the acoustic signals that corresponded to particular sounds would always be invariant. The task of speech production would be simplified if it were possible to produce an invariant acoustic signal without having to use precise articulatory maneuvers. The acoustic signals that correspond to various sounds are also more or less distinct from each other. The formant frequencies that specify the vowels [i] and [e] are, for example, closer to each other than the formant frequency patterns of [i] and [a] (Fant, 1960). The task of speech perception thus would also be made simpler if the acoustic signals that were used for vocal communication were maximally distinct. These criteria are captured by the physiological *quantal factor* introduced by Stevens (1972b).

The quantal factor can perhaps be illustrated by means of the following analogy. Suppose that an elegant restaurant is to open. The owner decides to employ waiters who will signal the diners' order by means of nonvocal acoustic signals. Shall he employ waiters equipped with violins or with sets of handbells? If he wants to minimize the chance of errors in communication he will opt for the handbells. Each bell produces a distinct acoustic signal without the waiters having to use precise manual gestures. In contrast, violins require comparatively precise maneuvers and will produce graded acoustic signals. The bells produce "quantal" signals, ones that yield distinct acoustic signals by means of relatively imprecise gestures.

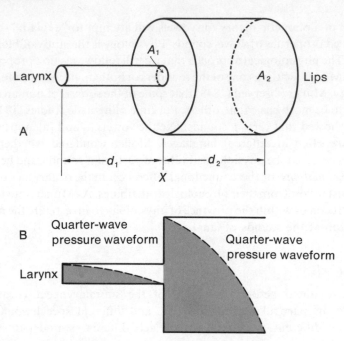

Figure 8.5. (A) Two-tube model of the supralaryngeal vocal tract for the vowel [a].
(B) Area function for two-tube model with air pressure waveforms sketched in.

Stevens (1972b) has demonstrated that certain speech sounds are more quantal than others. Vowels like [i], [u], and [a], for example, are specified by acoustic signals where formant frequencies converge. For [i] the second and third formants F_2 and F_3 are both high; [a] has a low F_2 and a high F_1; while [u] has a low F_1 and F_2. Distinct peaks in the spectrum of the acoustic signal automatically follow from these formant frequency convergences (Fant, 1956). In psychoacoustic tests involving English-speaking subjects the vowels [i] and [u] are more reliably identified than vowels like [ɪ], [e], or [ɛ] (Peterson and Barney, 1952; Fairbanks and Grubb, 1961). Stevens, by means of computer-implemented vocal modeling, demonstrated that these acoustic signals can be generated by means of relatively imprecise articulatory gestures.

In Figure 8.5A is sketched a stylized model of the cross-sectional area of the supralaryngeal vocal tract for the vowel [a]. The discussion that follows is essentially a paraphrase of Stevens' analysis (1972b). Stevens' insights on acoustic stability have provided a new way of looking at the nature of speech sounds. Note that the shape of the supralaryngeal vocal tract for this vowel approximates a two-tube resonator. The posterior portion of the supralaryngeal vocal tract, which corresponds to the pharynx, is constricted and has the cross-sectional area A_1. The anterior, oral cavity is relatively large.

The cross-sectional area of the oral cavity A_2 is about ten times as large as A_1 (Fant, 1960). To a first approximation the first two formant frequencies can be calculated as simple quarter-wavelength resonances of these two tubes. The discussion in Chapter 4 regarding the first resonance of a uniform tube applies to each tube because the coupling between the oral and pharyngeal tubes will be small as long as the cross-sectional areas A_1 and A_2 are substantially different.

The physical reasoning behind this approximation is not difficult to follow. At the closed end of the back tube, the air pressure that best "matches" the obstruction of the closed end is obviously a pressure maximum. The air pressure that best matches the end of the constricted tube at point X is zero pressure. This follows from the fact that the cross-sectional area A_2 is ten times greater than A_1. The size of the unconstricted tube is so much greater than that of the constricted tube to the outside atmosphere. A 10:1 difference in cross-sectional area is enormous. The effect on air pressure can be visualized by imagining what would happen to the members of a crowd as they exited from a passageway that was 3 feet wide to one 30 feet wide. The people in the crowd might be pushing against one another in the narrow passage. However, they could spread out in the 30 feet wide passage and never touch each other. The collision of the gas molecules that generated the air pressure waveform in the constricted tube is thus minimized at point X where the cross-sectional area abruptly changes. The air pressure waveform in the unconstricted tube is also a quarter-wave pattern, because the oral tube is nine-tenths "closed" at point X. The two pressure waveforms are sketched in Figure 8.5B.

The quarter-wave resonance model is only a first approximation to the behavior of the vocal tract for the vowel [a], e.g. the vowel of the word *hod*. It does, however, make evident the salient properties of this sound. The change in cross-sectional area, point X, occurs at the midpoint of the supralaryngeal vocal tract (Fant, 1960). F_1 and F_2, the first and second formant frequencies, are therefore, equal. If we perturbed the position of point X from this midpoint, we would not expect these two formant frequencies to change very abruptly. For example, if we moved point X 1 cm forward or backward we would generate the same first and second formant frequencies. The front tube would be longer and would generate the lower resonance F_1 if point X were moved 1 cm backward. If point X were instead moved 1 cm forward, the back cavity would generate the lower first formant. The first formant frequency would be identical for these two situations. It is immaterial whether the front or the back cavity generates the first formant frequency; all that matters is that the same frequency is generated. The second formant frequency would also have the same value for these two cases. It would be generated by the shorter tube. The first and second formant frequencies for the vowel [a] thus will not

173

change very much so long as point X is perturbed about the midpoint of the supralaryngeal vocal tract. An increase in the length of the front, oral cavity necessarily results in a decrease in the length of the back, pharyngeal cavity, and the two cavities "trade off" in generating the first and second formant frequencies.

The quarter-wave model for the vowel [a] is, as we have noted, a first approximation because there is actually some coupling between the front and back tubes. In Figure 8.6 calculated values for F_1 and F_2 are plotted for various positions of point X about the midpoint of a supralaryngeal vocal tract 17 cm long. These calculations were made using a computer-implemented model of the supralaryngeal vocal tract (Henke, 1966). The computer program calculates the formant frequencies of the supralaryngeal vocal tract for specified area functions. Note that the first and second formant frequencies converge for $X = 8.5$ cm, the midpoint of the supralaryngeal vocal tract. The quarter-wave approximation of [a] yields the same frequency for F_1 and F_2, but the coupling between the two tubes results in slightly different formant frequencies. Note that there is a range of about 2 cm in the middle of the curve of Figure 8.6 within which the second formant varies over only 50 Hz and the first formant changes even less. Within this region the two formants are close together. The transfer function for [a] in Figure 8.6 thus has a major spectral peak. In contrast, for the 2 cm range from $X = 11$ to 13 cm, the second formant frequency changes by about 0.4 kHz and the centered spectral peaks would be absent.

In Figure 8.7 illustrations of approximate midsagittal sections, cross-sectional area functions and acoustic transfer functions of the vocal tract for the vowels [i], [a] and [u] are presented. Articulatory and acoustic analyses have shown that these vowels are the limiting articulations of a vowel triangle that is language-universal (Trubetzkoy, 1939; Liljencrants and Lindblom, 1972). The body of the tongue is high and fronted to form a constricted oral cavity in [i], whereas it is low to form a large oral cavity in [a] and [u]. The pharynx is expanded in [i] and [u] and constricted in [a]. The oral and pharyngeal tubes are maximally expanded and/or maximally constricted in the production of these vowels. Further constriction would result in the generation of turbulent noise excitation and the loss of vowel quality (Fant, 1960; Stevens, 1972b).

Note that all three vowels have well-defined spectral properties. A central spectral peak occurs at about 1 kHz for [a]. A high frequency spectral peak occurs for [i] and a low frequency spectral peak occurs for [u]. More recent data indicate that listeners may use spectral information to assess vowel quality (Bladon and Lindblom, 1981). The converging formant frequencies of the quantal vowels inherently yield large spectral peaks; Fant (1956) demonstrated that a peak in the spectrum of a speech sound will occur whenever two

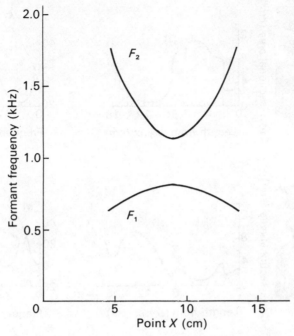

Figure 8.6. The first formant frequency F_1 *and the second formant frequency* F_2 *for the two-tube model of Figure 8.5. The formant frequencies were calculated using a computer model of the supralaryngeal vocal tract in which the position of the area function discontinuity, point* X, *was shifted forwards and backwards. (After Stevens, 1972b.)*

formant frequencies converge. The quantal vowels [i], [u] and [a] have well-defined spectral peaks because of the convergence of two formant frequencies. F_1 and F_2 converge to yield a central spectral peak at about 1 kHz for [a]. F_2 and F_3 converge to yield a high frequency peak for [i], F_1 and F_2 converge to yield a low frequency spectral peak for [u]. Psychoacoustic tests consistently show that the vowels [i] and [u] produce the fewest errors when listeners are asked to identify isolated vowels. The Peterson and Barney (1952) study of vowel acoustics and perception, for example, presented the vowels produced by 76 different speakers to a panel of listeners who were asked to identify the vowels. In any single trial the vowels of ten of the speakers were presented in random order so the listeners could not expect to hear either the voice of a particular speaker or a particular vowel. Under these conditions only ten misidentifications of [i] occurred in over 10 000 trials; 83 [u] errors occurred. The error rates for other vowels were about 8 percent. Similar results occurred in the experiments of Fairbanks and Grubb (1961), Bond (1976), Strange *et al.* (1976), Fowler and Shankweiler (1978), Pisoni, Carrell and Simnick (1979),

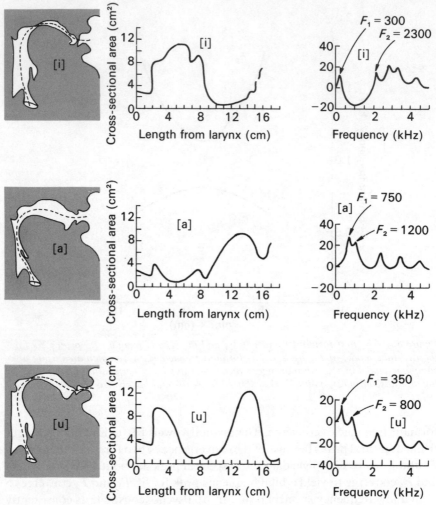

Figure 8.7. Midsagittal sections, cross-sectional area functions, and acoustic transfer functions of the vocal tract for the vowels [i], [a], and [u].

and Ryalls and Lieberman (1982). Surprisingly, high error rates occurred for [a], which we will discuss below.

Vocal tract normalization

The acoustic data of Peterson and Barney (1952) offer a clue to the high identification rates of the quantal vowels [i] and [u] and the misidentifications

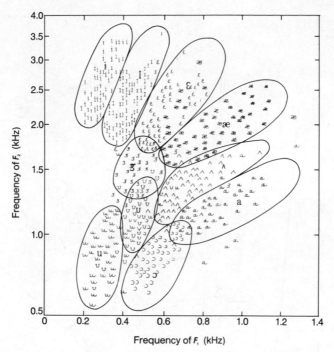

Figure 8.8. Classifying vowel sounds in terms of their first and second formant frequencies. Each letter represents a vowel that has F_1 *plotted on the abscissa (horizontal scale) and* F_2 *on the ordinate (vertical scale). (After Peterson and Barney, 1952.)*

that can occur for other vowels. They recorded a total of 76 adult male and female, and adolescent male and female speakers who each produced a series of English words of the form *head, heed, hid,* and so on. The word initial [h] resulted in noise excitation of the vowel that facilitated the measurement of formant frequencies from spectrograms. The plot in Figure 8.8 shows the frequencies of F_1 and F_2 for the individual vowel productions that each speaker intended as a token of an [i], [u], [e], etc. The loops on the plot enclose the vowel tokens that made up 90 percent of the tokens in each phonetic class. Note that there is overlap on the plot between tokens in adjacent phonetic categories. The data show that a sound intended by one speaker as an [ɛ] has the formant frequencies of another speaker's [ɪ]. The error patterns in the vowel identification test correspond to these overlaps. These overlaps occur, among other reasons, because different speakers have different supralaryngeal vocal tract lengths. Human speakers do not attempt to produce the same absolute formant frequency values for the "same" vowels. They instead

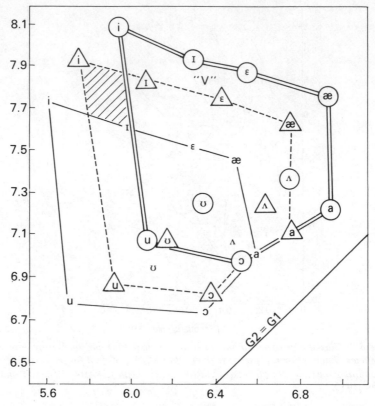

Figure 8.9. Average values of formant frequencies derived by Peterson and Barney for adult male speakers, adult female speakers (vowel points enclosed by triangles), and adolescents (vowel symbols enclosed by circles). The frequency values have been plotted on logarithmic scales. The vowel points of each class of speakers are connected and form relative vowel spaces. Note that the vowel spaces for the adult females and the adolescents are transposed upward in frequency from the vowel space of the adult males. (After Nearey, 1978.) From Lieberman, 1984.

produce a set of formant frequencies that is frequency-scaled to their approximate supralaryngeal vocal tract length.

The plot in Figure 8.9, which is from Nearey (1978), shows this effect more clearly. Nearey plotted the averages of the formant frequencies for F_1 and F_2 that Peterson and Barney (1952) derived for their adult male, adult female, and adolescent speakers. Nearey also converted the plots of formant frequencies to a logarithmic scale. Note that the shape of the vowel "space" is similar for the vowels of the three groups of speakers. The logarithmic plot allows us to see the similarity in shape that is preserved as the formant frequencies shift upwards from the values of the longer adult male supralaryngeal vocal tracts to the shorter adult female and adolescent supralaryngeal vocal tracts. The length of the supralaryngeal vocal tract does not reach its adult value until after puberty; adult women also tend to have shorter vocal tracts than do adult men (Goldstein, 1980). The quantal vowels [i], [u] and [a] and the vowel [æ], which forms a vowel "quadrilateral" in some languages (Trubetzkoy, 1939; Greenberg, 1963, 1966), define the vowel "space" within which the speakers differentiate the other vowels of English. Note that the [a] and [ɔ] points for the group averages of adolescents and adult males fall next to each other. A high rate of confusions occurs between [a] and [ɔ] in the Peterson and Barney (1952) data. These confusions are consistent with the instability of phonemic /a/ versus /ɔ/ distinctions in many dialects of English and other languages.

The errors in vowel perception that occurred in the Peterson and Barney (1952) data and in subsequent experiments occurred when listeners were uncertain about the identity of the speaker to whom they were listening. When different vowel tokens are "blocked" for each different speaker so that the listener hears one speaker at a time, these errors disappear (Strange *et al.*, 1976; Kahn, 1978; Assmann, 1979). These errors in vowel perception thus appear to follow from uncertainty regarding supralaryngeal vocal tract normalization. A human listener has to determine the probable length of the supralaryngeal vocal tract of the speakers he is listening to in order to determine the frequency parameters of the appropriate "vowel" space. Psychoacoustic experiments show that human listeners can make use of various acoustic cues and strategies to effect vocal tract normalization. The average level of formant frequencies of a short "carrier" phrase can for example, shift the perception of the vowel [ε] to [æ] or [ɪ] (Ladefoged and Broadbent, 1957). Ncarcy (1978) demonstrates that a token of the vowel [i] can shift the perception of the remainder of the vowel space of a listener. The vowel [i] is self-specifying for vocal tract length. The [i] vowels of different speakers form the extreme upper left margin of the vowel space plotted for different sized supralaryngeal vocal tracts. Thus a vowel having formant frequencies in this part of the vowel space must necessarily be a token of an [i].

In producing an [i], the tongue is moved upwards and forwards to such a degree that further movement in these directions would produce a constriction yielding air turbulence. The sound would no longer be a vowel, but instead would be a fricative, excited by noise generated at the constriction. The lack of overlap between [i] and other vowels in Figure 8.9 follows from the fact that the supralaryngeal vocal tract is pushed to its limit in producing an [i]. Unlike the other vowels, there is only one supralaryngeal vocal tract area function that can produce the formant frequency pattern of an [i]. This can be seen in the nomograms of Stevens and House (1955) and the computer modeling studies of Lieberman and Crelin (1971) and Lieberman, Crelin and Klatt (1972).

179

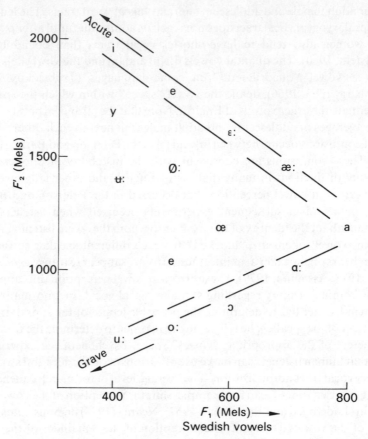

Figure 8.10. Acoustic classification of the vowels of Swedish in terms of Mel values of first formant and "equivalent" second formant frequencies. The acoustically defined phonetic features grave *and* acute *are used to differentiate these two classes of "peripheral" vowels.*

Consonants may also furnish cues for vocal tract normalization (Strange *et al.*, 1976). Human listeners probably adopt a strategy in which they make use of any cue that facilitates normalization.

The linguistic categorization of vowels

The data that we have discussed support the theory that was first proposed by Hellwag (1781). As Nearey (1978) demonstrates, Hellwag's vowel "diagram" categorizes vowels using a two-dimensional space that is roughly equivalent to the F_1 versus F_2 plot of Peterson and Barney (1952). In Figure 8.10 the frequency of the first formant of various vowels of Swedish are plotted with respect to the abscissa on a Mel scale. The "effective" second formant frequency is plotted with respect to the ordinate of Mels. The effective second formant frequency takes into account the spectral peaking effect that occurs when the second and third formant frequencies of a vowel approach each other. It thus yields a total spectrum that approximates the spectrum that would result if F_3 were represented when only F_1 and F_2 are used to synthesize a vowel. It therefore takes into account the perceptual effects of the higher formants (Fant, 1969).

The frequency values of these vowels are those derived by Fant (1969). The long vowels of Swedish are spaced out along the peripheral axis established by the vowels [i] and [a], and [u] and [a] in equal Mel intervals. This is in accord with the predictions of Lindblom (1971) regarding the preferred acoustic spacing of vowels along the peripheral axis established by the quantal vowels [i], [u] and [a]. These quantal vowels tend to occur more often in different languages (Trubetzkoy, 1939; Greenberg 1963, 1966); other vowels can occur in different languages if and only if these vowels also occur. The quantal vowels thus appear to be highly valued for speech communication. The term *markedness* was introduced by Trubetzkoy (1939) and Jakobson (1968) to convey the natural value of particular sounds. Sounds that are less marked are more prevalent and "natural" sounds. All other things being equal we would expect the least marked, i.e. the most highly valued and natural sounds, to occur most often in the inventory of sounds that occur in human languages. This, of course, does not mean that a particular language must make use of the most unmarked sounds. Human societies do not always make use of the simplest or most natural patterns of behavior. However, in a global sense we should expect to find the least marked sounds occurring most often.

All languages do not have the same inventory of peripheral, nonquantal vowels. In Figure 8.11 formant frequencies are plotted in Mels for the average values of the vowels of American English that were measured by Peterson and Barney (1952) and Potter and Steinberg (1950). Note that the [i] to [a] axis is divided up into the same set of vowels as Swedish (cf. Figure 8.10). Different symbols are used for the vowels of American English, and there may be differences in the lengths of some vowels between the two languages (e.g. [ɛ] and [ɛː]), but the formant frequency intervals are similar. The situation is quite different for the [u] to [a] axis. The vowels [o] and [oː] line up across the two languages, as do the vowels transcribed as [ɔ] in English and [ɑː] in Swedish. However, there is no vowel like Swedish [ɔ] in English. The Swedish [uː] is likewise different from English [u]. These differences point out the dangers of relying too heavily on phonetic studies that compare the sounds of different languages without making use of objective acoustic analysis.

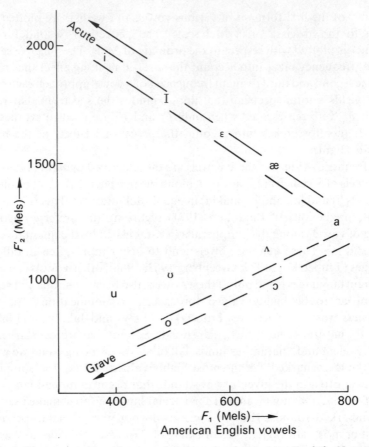

Figure 8.11. Acoustic classification of the vowels of American English. Note that the distribution of vowels is different and that the "same" phonetic symbol, e.g. [ɔ], has different acoustic values in the Swedish than in the American English data.

Psychoacoustic data (Stevens, Liberman and Studdert-Kennedy, 1969) indicate that monolingual speakers of American English are not able to identify the Swedish vowels [y] and [ʉː] with certainty. Swedish listeners, as we might expect, are able to identify these vowels with certainty. What might the psychological basis for these different vowel distinctions be? The only plausible hypothesis appears to be one that involves either a universal set of neural property detectors that are selectively activated as people are exposed to particular sounds during a "plastic" period, or a completely plastic process that "shapes up" property detectors for sounds used in the language. In short, vowels seem to be perceived by means of neural acoustic property detectors that respond to particular acoustic signals. Thus acoustic rather than articulatory factors specify vowels. The range of formant frequencies to which these property detectors can potentially respond, however, is delimited by the quantal vowels [i], [u] and [a]. The acoustic properties of these vowels reflect the constraints of the species-specific supralaryngeal vocal tract anatomy of *Homo sapiens*, which we will discuss in Chapter 9. Like the bullfrogs which we discussed in Chapter 7, we seem to respond to particular vowel sounds by means of neural devices that are "tuned" to particular acoustic signals that reflect the constraints of our speech producing mechanisms. Humans however, unlike frogs, are plastic and will partition the possible range of formant frequencies that the human vocal tract can generate differently, as they grow up in different linguistic environments.

Phonetic features

The challenge for any phonetic theory is not only to account for the nature of human speech sounds, their production and perception, but also to explain how speech sounds function in language. For example, English has in its inventory of sounds, only a small subset of the possible speech sounds in natural language. While we may have stop consonants in which the closure is at the lips [p b], alveolar ridge [t d], or velum [k g], we do not have stop consonants where the closure is made on the hard palate. In contrast, Russian does have such sounds. Nevertheless, linguists such as Roman Jakobson observed that despite the fact that languages may have a different array of sounds, there are not only certain regularities within any one language, but more interestingly, there are certain regularities among *all* the languages of the world. Jakobson proposed that the speech sounds occurring in the languages of the world could be described in terms of a finite set of attributes called *phonetic features* (Jakobson, Fant and Halle, 1963; Jakobson and Waugh, 1979). For example, the sound [p] can be further analyzed as a consonant [+ consonantal], it is produced with a full stop or closure [+ stop], the closure is at the lips [+ labial], and the vocal cords are delayed in vibrating until about 20 milliseconds after the release of the stop closure [− voice]. Further, he proposed that all of the speech sounds occurring in natural language can be described with only 12 or so phonetic features.

Linguists have long noted the importance of phonetic features in describing the sound structure of language and in postulating how the sound systems of language change (Chomsky and Halle, 1968). In fact, as early as about 600 BC, Pāṇini, the great Indian grammarian, implicitly recognized the phonetic feature in his analysis of the sound structure of Sanskrit. And psycholinguists have shown that the phonetic feature seems to be a basic processing unit in speech production and speech perception. Evidence from "slips of the tongue" produced by normal subjects, for example, shows that phonetic features and segments are planning units for speech production (Fromkin, 1971, 1973). As we shall describe in Chapter 9, many of the speech production impairments of aphasic patients can be characterized in terms of the substitution of one phonetic feature for another. As to perception, Miller and Nicely (1955) analyzed the errors that English-speaking listeners made when they identified consonant–vowel syllables mixed with noise or filtered. The noise and filtering made the listeners' task more difficult and it threw into relief effects that might not otherwise be evident. Sounds were confused in consistent patterns which corresponded to misperceptions of a single phonetic feature. For example, the sounds [p], [t], [k], as a class, were confused with the sounds [b], [d], [g]. The first group shares the phonetic feature [−voiced], and the second group the feature [+voiced]. Moreover, normal subjects take a longer time to discriminate sounds distinguished by one phonetic feature, e.g. [p] vs. [b], than sounds distinguished by more than one phonetic feature, e.g. [p] vs. [d] (Baker, Blumstein and Goodglass, 1981).

Jakobson postulated that phonetic features could be defined in reference to acoustic patterns or acoustic properties derivable from the speech signal. That is, for each phonetic feature there was a hypothesized corresponding acoustic property. These properties were defined in terms of spectral patterns or changes in the overall amplitude characteristics of the speech signal. Unlike the motor theory of speech which we discussed earlier, for Jakobson, the acoustic signal was paramount since "... we speak to be heard in order to be understood" (Jakobson, Fant and Halle, 1963, p.13).

Nevertheless, what is not explained by Jakobson's theory is *why* there are a finite number of features, and *why* the particular features and their corresponding acoustic properties take the particular form that they do. One recent theory has suggested that the answers to these questions have to do with the physiological constraints imposed on the human vocal apparatus, on the one hand, and the human auditory system, on the other. In this view, it is proposed that the physiological constraints provide, as it were, the defining characteristics for the particular sound shape of natural language. Let us briefly explore this theory.

Physiological constraints

It is obvious that the articulatory and auditory systems have certain intrinsic limits, i.e. a sound cannot be produced if it is beyond the physiological capacity of the production system, and it cannot be perceived if its characteristics fall out of the range of the auditory system. Thus, no language has a speech sound produced with the tongue tip tapping the point of the nose, and no language has a sound which has a frequency of 100 000 Hz. However, the sounds of

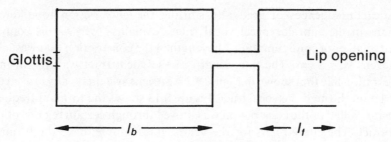

Figure 8.12. An idealized model of the supralaryngeal vocal tract for the production of fricative consonants. The position of the constriction can be shifted by changing the values of the length of the back and front cavities, l_b *and* l_f.

language seem to be constrained by physiological factors in even more fundamental and interesting ways. It has been suggested that physiological constraints on both the human vocal tract and the auditory system provide a limiting condition on the particular sound shape of language.

Let us first consider possible articulatory constraints. Stevens' quantal theory, which we have already discussed for vowels, lays the foundation for the constraints on the articulatory system as they influence the sound shape of language. While, in principle, there are a potentially infinite number of places of articulation, languages of the world seem to make use of at most seven different places of articulation, and no language uses all seven of these (Ladefoged, 1971; Greenberg, 1963, 1966). Why? As we have noted above, Stevens has shown that there are certain articulatory regions called *quantal regions* for which distinctive acoustic patterns result. Within these regions, small articulatory changes do not significantly affect the acoustic patterns. As a result, in these regions, less articulatory precision is required in order to produce the same acoustic pattern. These regions are called quantal because within the region small articulatory changes have minimal acoustic effects, whereas at the boundaries of these regions, articulatory changes of the same magnitude will result in significant changes in the acoustic pattern. Stevens points out that the stable acoustic patterns generated within the quantal regions furthermore can be characterized by well-defined spectral peaks.

In Figure 8.12, an idealized model for the production of a fricative consonant is shown. The glottis is at the left-hand end of the tube and is considered to be almost closed. The position of the constriction, which is between l_b and l_f, can be adjusted to represent different places of articulation. From a simple-minded articulatory point of view there is no reason why a constriction could not be formed at any point in the supralaryngeal vocal tract from the lips down to the pharynx. In fact, this is precisely what occurs when you swallow food. The food is pushed back along the supralaryngeal vocal tract by the tongue and pharyngeal constrictures. Stevens' modeling of the acoustic consequences of gradually shifting the constriction to different positions in the supralaryngeal vocal tract "explains" why we use only a limited number of configurations. The length of the constriction that was used by Stevens was 3 cm. The total length of the vocal tract was 16 cm in a configuration like that shown in Figure 8.12. Stevens systematically moved the constriction through the vocal tract. Figure 8.13 shows the formant frequencies that resulted as the constriction was moved through certain regions of the vocal tract. The curved bars for the velars, for example, have the formant frequencies that resulted when the constriction was such that the length of the back cavity (as shown in Figure 8.12) was between 8.0 and 9.8 cm.

The curved "bars" on Figure 8.13 indicate the quantal acoustic signals that result as particular formant frequencies generated by the front and back cavities, l_f and l_b, couple to produce spectral peaks and relative insensitivity to small articulatory perturbations in the two pharyngeal articulations ($l_b = 5$ and 7 cm), the velar articulation ($l_b = 9$ cm), the retroflex articulation, produced with the tip of the tongue curled back, ($l_b = 10$ cm), and the dental articulation ($l_b = 11$ cm). The labial articulation which occurs for $l_b = 13$ cm always results in formant frequencies lower than the formant frequencies of the unconstricted vocal tract. Thus the formant frequencies of a vowel–labial consonant sequence will always involve falling transitions. The acoustic signals that specify the pharyngeal points of articulation are shaded in this diagram since these consonants involving these regions do not occur in English and their acoustic properties have not been studied extensively.

The sketch derived from lateral X-ray views in Figure 8.13B shows the labial, dental and velar articulations. There may be minor differences between different speakers and different languages. Stevens' model is oversimplified, but it points out the salient quantal properties of the different phonetic features relevant for describing place of articulation.

In order for languages to use phonetic categories in speech, it is necessary to have a distinctive acoustic pattern to define that category so that the listener can perceive it, and it is useful that the articulatory system can produce this pattern even with some articulatory imprecision. Thus, while in principle there should be a potentially infinite number of phonetic categories which can be produced by the vocal tract, the quantal nature of speech production severely limits the total number of potential phonetic categories.

Just as the articulatory system has fundamental constraints, so does the auditory system. As we discussed earlier, both infants and adults hear speech continua in a categorical fashion. These observations about categorical perception suggest that there are perceptual limitations on the possible number of speech sounds that can occur in language.

If we consider the articulatory constraints postulated by the quantal theory

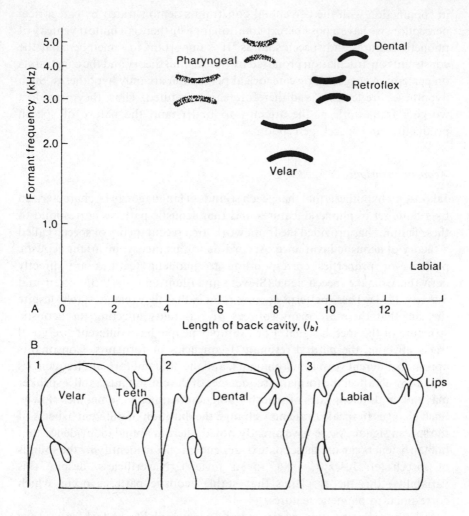

Figure 8.13. (A) Results of a computer modeling of the model of Figure 8.12. The curved bars indicate the quantal acoustic signals that are produced at particular "points of articulation." (B) Sketches of supralaryngeal vocal tract for labial, dental, and velar stops (the stop sounds [p], [t] and [k]). The retroflex and pharyngeal quantal regions shown in Figure 8.13 (A) are not used in English.

in conjunction with the perceptual constraints demonstrated by categorical perception, we have a possible explanation for *why* there is a finite inventory of phonetic features and speech sounds. It is important to remember that the constraints on articulation proposed by the quantal theory and the constraints on perception suggested by categorical perception are only hypotheses. Such hypotheses are testable, and therefore can be refuted. Thus, they provide a working framework in the attempt to understand the nature of speech production and speech perception.

Acoustic invariance in speech

Jakobson's hypothesis that the speech sounds of language can be characterized by a finite set of phonetic features and that acoustic patterns correspond to these features has provided the framework for a recent theory of speech called a theory of acoustic invariance. According to this theory, invariant acoustic patterns or properties corresponding to phonetic features are directly derivable from the speech signal (Stevens and Blumstein, 1981; Blumstein and Stevens, 1981). These patterns are invariant in that they remain stable despite the fact that there are many sources of variability affecting the acoustic structure of the speech signal. For example, people have different size vocal tracts affecting the natural resonant frequencies or formants. Consonants appear in different vowel environments, and the different formant frequencies of the vowels affect the formant frequencies of the consonants. And a speaker may talk at different rates of speech – sometimes quickly, sometimes slowly. Such changes in speaker rate may change the duration of different aspects of the speech signal. As we have already noted, there is abundant evidence that human listeners can use these context-dependent cues in identifying the sounds of speech (cf. Jusczyk, 1986, for a review). Nevertheless, despite this variability, this theory claims that stable acoustic patterns occur which correspond to phonetic features.

If there are invariant properties, what do they look like and where are they found? This search for acoustic invariance can be guided by two considerations. First, what articulatory states are least likely to be affected by sources of acoustic variation, either due to phonetic context as the articulatory structures are in transition from one target configuration to another, or due to individual vocal tract sizes and shapes affecting the natural frequencies for a given sound? Second, what are the response characteristics of the auditory system to speech-like sounds? In other words what are likely to be acoustically stable properties, both articulatorily and perceptually?

Several researchers exploring these questions have investigated whether invariant properties corresponding particularly to consonants reside where

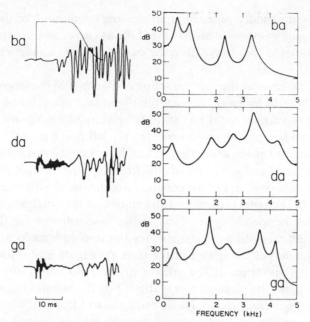

Figure 8.14. Examples of waveforms and spectra at the release of three voiced stop consonants as indicated. From Stevens and Blumstein, 1981.

there are rapid spectral or amplitude changes within a fairly short time domain (Searle, Jacobson and Rayment, 1979; Stevens and Blumstein, 1981; Kewley-Port, 1983). These regions correspond to the tens of milliseconds in the vicinity of the consonantal release. At these points in time, the articulators may be least affected by the transition from one articulatory state to the other, i.e. phonetic context. The types of patterns likely to contain acoustic invariance are postulated by these researchers to be generalized patterns in the frequency/amplitude domain, ie. spectral patterns, which will not be dependent upon details of the fine acoustic structure such as the absolute formant frequencies.

These generalized patterns are called *integrated* acoustic properties because they encompass several components of the acoustic signal including the relative distribution of the formant frequency peaks, the relation among the amplitudes of the frequency peaks, and/or the change in the spectral or amplitude distribution over a short time period. For example, invariant properties have been proposed for place of articulation in stop consonants. These properties correspond to the gross shape of the spectrum sampled at the release of the stop consonant. They incorporate spectral information of the burst as well as some tens of milliseconds of the formant transitions. Figure 8.14 shows how the stimuli are analyzed. On the left are the waveform displays for the syllables [ba], [da] and [ga]. The burst can be seen, particularly for [da] and [gɑ], by the sudden onset of rapid random fluctuations of the waveform display. The quasi-periodic display that follows corresponds to the motion of the articulators as they move from the closure into the configuration for the vowel.

In order to see what the spectral shape of the onset of the stop is, i.e. to see not only where the formant peaks are relative to each other, but also how large they are, it is essential to take a "still-life" picture of a portion of the signal. Thus, a window is placed, as shown in the top left panel, over the burst. Note that the window encompasses about 25 milliseconds of the speech signal, and includes the burst and some tens of milliseconds of the formant transitions. A linear predictive coding (LPC) is conducted of the signal within the window of analysis. On the right is displayed the results of this analysis, showing the spectrum of the speech signal. Time in this case is frozen for the spectrum represents the integration of the frequency and amplitude peaks within the first 25.6 milliseconds of the release of the stop. As Figure 8.14 shows, the gross shape of the spectrum at the release of the stop consonant is different depending upon the place of articulation. For the labial consonant [b], the peaks in the spectrum are, as Jakobson, Fant and Halle (1963) noted, fairly spread out or *diffuse*, and there is greater spectral energy in the lower frequencies than in the higher frequencies. This spectrum shape is described as *diffuse-falling*. For the alveolar stop [d], the spectral peaks are also diffuse, but the amplitudes of these peaks are greater in the higher frequencies. This spectrum shape is described as *diffuse-rising*. And although there are a number of peaks in the spectrum for the velar consonant [g], there is one spectral peak dominating the entire spectrum. Following Jakobson, the spectrum shape is described as *compact*.

These patterns occur for both voiced and voiceless labial, alveolar and velar consonants as they occur in different vowel environments and as they are produced by different speakers (Stevens and Blumstein, 1979; Blumstein and Stevens, 1979, 1981). The patterns emerge most clearly when the consonant appears in initial position. But they also occur when the consonant appears in final position, if it is released. Other researchers (Searle, Jacobson and Rayment 1979; Kewley-Port, 1983), using slightly different measurement procedures, have also found invariant patterns corresponding to place of articulation in initial position for English stop consonants.

Listeners also seem to be sensitive to the information present in the onset spectrum. In several studies (Blumstein and Stevens, 1980; Kewley-Port, Pisoni and Studdert-Kennedy, 1983), subjects were presented with a series of synthetic stimuli appropriate to the consonants [b d g] in the environment of the vowels [i a u]. Figure 8.15 shows how the stimuli were constructed. These

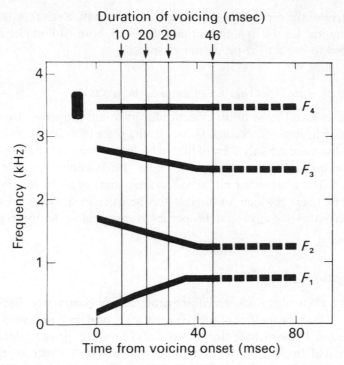

Figure 8.15. Schematized spectrographic representation of a stimulus with formant trajectories appropriate for the syllable [da]. From Blumstein and Stevens, 1980.

stimuli contain the stop burst followed by the first 5, 10, 20 or 40 milliseconds of the formant transitions. One group of listeners was asked to identify the consonant, and another group was asked to identify the vowel. Results showed that listeners were able to identify the correct place of articulation for the stop consonant. In addition, they could also identify the correct vowel. These results show that the onset properties can be used by the listener to differentiate components of the consonant–vowel syllable relating to consonant place of articulation and to vowel quality. And this information is available in the absence of full formant transitions and steady-state vowel information.

Even infants can discriminate these onset properties (Bertoncini *et al.*, 1987). Three- and four-day-old infants were presented with a subset of the stimuli given to the adults. They were given the stimuli which contained the burst and the first 20 milliseconds of the formant transitions. Using a nonnutritive sucking paradigm (see Chapter 9), it was found that they could not only discriminate place of articulation, but they could also discriminate vowel quality. Thus, from birth, infants behave similar to adults. They seem to

191

be sensitive to the rapid changes in the onset spectrum. Such results provide strong support for the hypothesis that infants are born with innate mechanisms tuned to extract the properties of speech.

Invariant acoustic properties for other phonetic features

We have reviewed some of the evidence for invariant properties for place of articulation in stop consonants. However, the place of articulation contrasts we have discussed are only a few of the twelve or so phonetic features proposed by Jakobson (Jakobson, Fant and Halle, 1963) comprising the speech inventory. There are other phonetic features, some of them relating to the different manners in which consonants may be articulated. Let us review some of the hypothesized invariant properties corresponding to these phonetic features.

Abrupt–continuant

There is a class of sounds which are produced by completely blocking the airstream along the midline of the laryngeal and vocal tract pathways prior to their release. These include stop consonants [p t k b d g], affricates [č ǰ] and nasals [m n ŋ]. In contrast, there is another class of sounds which are produced by a constriction in the vocal tract without completely blocking the airstream. These include the glides [w y] and the fricatives [f θ s š v δ z ž]. Invariant acoustic properties have been proposed to distinguish the class of abrupt consonants from continuant consonants (Stevens and Blumstein, 1981; Mack and Blumstein, 1983). These properties correspond to changes in the amplitude characteristics of the signal. For abrupt consonants, there is a rapid change in amplitude in the vicinity of the consonant release, and this rapid amplitude increase occurs in all frequencies. For continuant consonants, there is a more gradual change in the vicinity of the release, particularly in the mid and high frequencies.

Let us compare the stop [b] and the glide [w] to illustrate this contrast. The stop [b] is produced with a complete closure at the lips followed by a release of the closure as the articulators move into the configuration for the following vowel. As a result of the closure, there is an increase in air pressure behind the constriction, and at the moment of consonant release, there is an abrupt and transient increase in sound pressure. The acoustic consequence of such articulatory maneuvers is a rapid rise of acoustic energy at the release of the stop. In contrast, the glide [w] is produced with a partial constriction in the vocal tract, and there is a more gradual release of the articulators into the configuration for the following vowel. As a result, there is only a small rise in air pressure owing to the partial constriction, and there is a gradual increase in sound pressure. The acoustic property resulting from these articulatory gestures is a gradual rise of acoustic energy at the release of the glide. Figure 8.16 shows the difference in the amplitude properties of the stop [b] and the glide [w]. This figure shows a frequency–amplitude–time display of the syllables [bi] and [wi]. A series of LPC analyses are done, placing a 25.6 millisecond window prior to the consonant release and moving this window in 5 millisecond steps through the release of the consonant and into the following vowel. This figure then provides a three-dimensional display of the amplitude and spectral changes charted over time. The large and abrupt changes in amplitude for the stop [b] between 37 and 75 milliseconds compared to the more gradual changes in amplitude for the glide [w] are readily apparent in Figure 8.16. Note that the abrupt changes in amplitude for the stop occur in all frequency regions, as does the gradual increase in energy for the glide.

Fricative consonants are also continuants. Unlike the abrupt, noncontinuant consonants which show a rapid amplitude change in all frequencies, the fricative consonant [s], like the glide [w], shows gradual amplitude changes, particularly in the mid and high frequencies.

Perception studies have shown that listeners seem to be sensitive to the acoustic properties described above in perceiving the contrast between abrupt consonants and continuant consonants. In one experiment, stimuli with an abrupt rise in amplitude at the consonant release were perceived as stops, e.g. [b], while stimuli with a gradual rise at the consonant release were perceived as continuants, e.g. [v] or [w] (Shinn and Blumstein, 1984). In another experiment, it was shown that the continuant [š], for which the onset amplitude is rather gradual, is perceived as the affricate [č], an abrupt consonant, when the initial part of the frication noise is removed, leaving an abrupt amplitude rise in the noise (Cutting and Rosner, 1974; Cutting, 1982).

Nasal–nonnasal
As we have described in the previous section, nasal consonants as [m n ŋ] have an abrupt onset, because of the complete closure in the oral cavity. However, for nasals, there is an additional invariant property, corresponding to the phonetic feature [nasal]. This property is associated with the presence of a murmur in the vicinity of the consonant release. The acoustic property of a murmur is a broad resonant peak around 250 Hz with other resonant peaks lower in amplitude occurring above 700 Hz. This murmur must occur in the closure interval preceding the consonant release. Nasalization may also continue into the vowel transitions immediately after the release of the closure until the velopharyngeal port is closed.

Perception studies have shown that for a consonant to be perceived as a

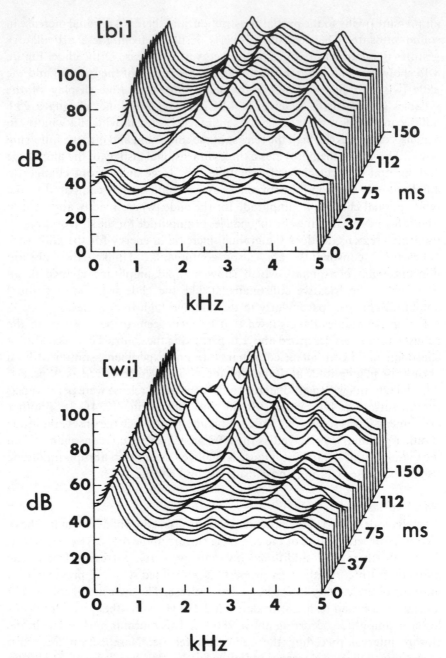

Figure 8.16. Three-dimensional frequency, amplitude and time display of [bi] and [wi]. The consonantal release in both utterances is located at 50 milliseconds. From Mack and Blumstein, 1983.

194

nasal, a murmur must occur in the closure interval. If it does not, the consonant is heard as a stop (Kurowski and Blumstein, 1984; Repp, 1986). This murmur may be very short in duration, as little as two glottal pulses. Moreover, there may need to be some nasalization in the vowel transitions as well. Otherwise, the consonant will not be heard as a true nasal (Katz and Blumstein, 1987). The spectral properties of the murmur are critical for the perception of nasal consonants. It is not the case that any appreciable energy occurring in the closure interval will serve as a cue to nasality. Rather, as described above, there needs to be a broad resonance peak around 250 Hz, and higher resonant peaks may need to be present as well.

Voiced–voiceless
Many languages of the world distinguish voiced segments from voiceless ones. In English, for example, the consonants [p t k f s] are voiceless and the consonants [b d g v z] are voiced. The acoustic property corresponding to the feature voiced is the presence of low frequency spectral energy or periodicity due to the vibration of the vocal cords. Voiceless sounds do not have such periodicity. The presence of this low frequency periodicity occurs for consonant sounds over a time interval of 20–30 milliseconds in the vicinity of the acoustic discontinuity that precedes or follows the consonant constriction interval (cf. Stevens and Blumstein, 1981; Lisker and Abramson, 1964).

Nevertheless, a number of researchers have suggested that there are other acoustic cues besides low frequency periodicity which also contribute to the voiced–voiceless contrast. Among these cues are the frequency of the first formant at the onset of voicing (Stevens and Klatt, 1974), the nature of the fundamental frequency f_0 changes immediately following consonant release (Haggard, Ambler and Callow, 1970), the frequency of the burst and the second and higher formants (Abramson and Lisker, 1970), the intensity of aspiration noise relative to the vowel (Repp, 1979), the duration of a preceding vowel (Denes, 1955; Klatt, 1973; Summerfield, 1975). This "many-to-one mapping," i.e. many acoustic cues signalling one phonetic dimension (Lisker *et al.*, 1977), provides a challenge for those searching for a single invariant property corresponding to one phonetic feature, since these data suggest that there is not always one simple invariant property corresponding to the phonetic feature for voicing. However, the multiple acoustic cues that signal voicing all appear to follow from the articulatory maneuvers that initiate voicing and may reflect a more complex "integrated" property detector that has evolved to facilitate the perception of human speech. However, much more research will be required to determine whether such a property can be discovered.

It is worth considering the feature *voicing* in more detail to illustrate that

195

phonetic features have both an articulatory basis, as they are produced by the vocal tract, and an acoustic basis, as they provide relevant perceptual attributes for distinguishing the sound contrasts occurring in language.

The activity of the muscles of the larynx is independent of the muscles that can open your lips or move your tongue when you produce a stop consonant like [b], [p] or [d]. The articulatory activity of the supralaryngeal vocal tract is independent of the larynx and is identical for the labial stop consonants [b] and [p] produced in similar contexts, e.g. the words *bat* and *pat*. What is different is the activity of the laryngeal muscles with respect to the abrupt lip opening that marks the start of the initial sound in both of these words. In both words, the audible acoustic signal commences at the instant when the speaker's lips open. In the case of the word *bat* the speaker's larynx is already in its closed, phonatory position at the moment that the speaker opens his lips. The vocal cords have already moved into their closed, or nearly closed, position and phonation is a consequence of the air flow through the vocal tract. High-speed movies of the larynx show that phonation starts about 10 to 20 milliseconds after the start of air flow if the vocal cords are already in their "phonation neutral" position (Lieberman, 1967). When the lips open in the word *bat*, air can flow through the vocal tract and phonation starts shortly thereafter.

In the word *pat* the situation is different. The vocal cords are still open at the instant the speaker's lips open. The sound that initially occurs is not voiced since phonation cannot occur when the vocal cords are open. The open position of the vocal cords instead allows a relatively large air flow and the initial sound is generated by the air turbulence that occurs as the lips are abruptly opened. An initial "burst" of air, therefore, can occur when a [p] is produced, particularly when it occurs in initial position. The speaker producing the word *pat* starts to close his vocal cords after the release of the [p]. The distinction between [b] and [p] thus rests on the delay in the start of phonation relative to the opening of the speaker's lips.

Phonation onset or voice-onset time (VOT), which we illustrated with an example drawn from English, simply involves the timing between the onset of phonation and the release of the primary occlusion of the vocal tract. Phonation onset as we have just described is relevant only for stop consonants, since only stop consonants have a full occlusion in the oral cavity. Nevertheless, the presence of low frequency periodicity in the vicinity of the consonant release provides the relevant acoustic attributes for the phonetic feature of voicing in all consonant sounds.

When a stop consonant occurs in initial position in the production of an isolated syllable, phonation can start coincident with the release of the stop, after the release of the stop, or before the release of the primary occlusion. In English the sound [p] is produced with *delayed* phonation. The sound [b] in

English is produced either with *coincident* or *advanced* phonation. In many languages the *advanced* versus *coincident* contrast is the relevant phonemic distinction (e.g. Spanish). In some languages all three categories are phonemic (e.g. Thai). The exact time intervals that characterize these categories vary from language to language (Lisker and Abramson, 1964, 1971). However, three categories potentially exist.

The perceptual responses of human listeners to voicing in stop consonants bears close inspection, for it reveals a fundamental underlying biological mechanism that structures this phonetic feature. If a large number of examples of the production of the English stops [p] and [b] are measured, it becomes evident that there is a good deal of variation in the timing between the onset of phonation and the release of the stop. Some [b]s have a phonation delay of 10 milliseconds, others 20 milliseconds and so on. Some [p]s have phonation delays of 50 milliseconds, others 60 milliseconds, others 40 milliseconds. The perceptual responses of listeners to these stimuli show categorical perception; namely listeners categorically perceive phonation onset or voice-onset time. They can only discriminate reliably those stimuli which they identify as belonging to different phonetic categories, i.e. voiced and voiceless, and their discrimination functions are "sharp" (cf. Chapter 7). Stops that have phonation delays less than 25 milliseconds are perceived as [b]. Stops that have phonation delays greater than 25 milliseconds are perceived as [p]. The situation is seemingly odd because these same listeners cannot perceive any difference between versions of [p] that differ as much as 20 milliseconds in their phonation delay. For example, listeners are not able to discriminate between two sounds that have phonation delays of 40 and 60 milliseconds respectively. But if the phonation delay of two sounds are 10 and 30 milliseconds, one sound will be heard and identified as [b], the other as [p]. In other words, listeners cannot differentiate sounds within each phonetic category although they sharply differentiate stimuli across the phonetic boundary on the basis of the same physical parameter, the 20 millisecond timing distinction. These distinctions occur across many related and unrelated languages (Lisker and Abramson, 1964). The basis of the 20 millisecond timing distinction appears to rest in a basic constraint of the auditory system. Hirsch (1959) and Hirsch and Sherrick (1961) carried out a series of experiments to determine the difference in time that is required for a listener to judge which of two auditory stimuli with diverse characteristics came first. A time difference of 20 milliseconds was found to be necessary for a variety of stimulus conditions.

The phonetic feature *voicing* thus appears to be inherently structured in terms of this perceptual constraint as well as the articulatory constraints of the speech-producing apparatus. The control of the source of excitation for speech is independent of the configuration of the supralaryngeal vocal tract. Speakers can thus change the timing between the laryngeal source and the opening of the supralaryngeal vocal tract. The magnitude of the time interval that differentiates the categories seems to be a consequence of the minimum temporal resolution of the auditory system.

The 20 millisecond timing distinction has been shown to mark the perception of stop sounds by one-month-old infants (Eimas *et al.*, 1971). Experiments monitoring their behavior while they listen to artificially synthesized stimuli have shown that they partition the temporal variations that can occur between phonation and the release of the primary occlusion of the supralaryngeal vocal tract at precisely the same 20 millisecond intervals used by normal adults and older children. There seems to be no way in which one month-old infants could "learn" to respond to speech stimuli in this manner. The 20 millisecond voicing onset interval appears to reflect an innately determined constraint of the auditory system in *Homo sapiens*.

Studies of the responses of chinchillas (Kuhl and Miller, 1971) to stop consonants show that these animals also are sensitive to the same 20 millisecond threshold. The animals can be taught to discriminate the sound [d] from [t] and their responses appear to be structured by the same 20 millisecond "temporal resolving" factor that operates in humans. This result is, of course, what we would expect if human language and human speech were the result of a gradual Darwinian process of evolution (Lieberman, 1975) and if the human speech apparatus were "built" on the capacities of the mammalian auditory system.

Prosodic features

Variations of stress and intonation convey both linguistic and "paralinguistic" or "emotional" information (Scherer, 1981). We discussed some of the acoustic correlates and articulatory maneuvers that manifest and generate the prosodic feature *stress* in Chapter 6. Variations in stress (Daniel Jones (1932) used the term *prominence*) have systematic linguistic functions in many languages and the acoustic correlates and underlying physiology have been carefully investigated in many experiments, e.g. Fry (1955), Lieberman (1960, 1967), Lehiste (1961), Morton and Jassem (1965), Atkinson (1973). We would have to list about 100 references if we wanted to present a comprehensive listing of recent work. *Tone* features which play an important linguistic role in many languages other than English, for example, Swedish and Thai, have also been carefully studied (Garding, Fujimura and Hirose, 1970; Erikson, 1975). In Chinese, for example, two words may differ phonetically solely with respect to the tone pattern of fundamental frequency. The study of these "tone" languages reveals that speakers execute deliberate laryngeal maneuvers to produce consistent f_0 contours (Erikson, 1975). There is, however, a second, more general function of the temporal pattern of fundamental frequency that is structured with regard to the biological constraints of respiration. The pattern of fundamental frequency plays a role in signaling the end of a sentence in most, if not all, human languages (Lieberman, 1967; Vanderslice and Ladefoged, 1972). Both traditional and generative grammars (Chomsky, 1957) regard a sentence as the minimal unit from which a complete semantic interpretation can be made. The traditional functional description of a sentence, that it expresses a complete thought, has real validity. It is easy to perform a small experiment that tests this statement. All that one has to do is read a short passage after moving the sentence-final period punctuation one word over. The resulting sequences of words will, for the most part, be unintelligible. The primary function of orthographic punctuation is to indicate the ends of sentences. The sentence-final "period" symbol is essential. Question marks can be optionally replaced by special words in most languages. (English is a special case in so far as some of the options have fallen out of use in comparatively recent times (cf. Lieberman, 1967)). Commas are usually optional in so far as the reader would have been able to derive the sentence's meaning if they were omitted. During normal speech the prosodic content of the message, which is largely determined by the perceived pitch as a function of time, signals the ends of sentences. The phonetic feature that speakers make use of to segment the train of words into sentences is the *breath-group*.

The breath-group as a phonetic feature has a long history. It derives from the "tune" analysis of Armstrong and Ward (1926) and Jones (1932). Stetson (1951) introduced the concept of a physiologically structured basic prosodic signal. The breath-group is a central, basic aspect of language since it signals phonetically the boundaries of sentences. It is not a question of language being more difficult to comprehend without signaling the boundaries of sentences. Language would be difficult if not impossible without this information, for we would be reduced to one-word utterances, each of which would have a fixed, immutable meaning. Language is not a code in which particular signals have fixed meanings. Language has the potential of transmitting new, unanticipated information. Syntax and the sentence are necessary factors for the presence of language, and the breath-group is one of the basic, primitive phonetic features that serves as an organizing principle for these factors.

This view of the basic, primitive status of the breath-group is consistent with the physiological mechanisms that structure and constrain its form. In the production of normal speech the acoustic cues that characterize the normal breath-group are a consequence of minimal deviation from the respiratory activity that is necessary to sustain life. The primary function of the human respiratory system is *not* to provide air for speech production. Oxygen transfer to the blood stream is the primary vegetative function of the respiratory system. Speech production is a secondary function. Constant respiratory activity is necessary to sustain life, and in the absence of speech there is an ongoing cyclic pattern in which inspiration is followed by expiration as the lungs alternately expand and deflate, forcing air in and out through the nose, mouth, pharynx and trachea. In Chapter 6 graphs of pulmonary air pressure were presented for both quiet respiration and speech (Figure 6.1). Similar data have been derived for various types of utterances and the details of the pulmonary air pressure function vary. However, one factor is always present. The pulmonary air pressure during the expiratory phase must be greater than the atmospheric air pressure. During the inspiratory phase it must, in contrast, be lower than the atmospheric air pressure. At the end of the expiratory phase of the breath-group, there must be a fairly abrupt transition in the pulmonary air pressure from the greater (positive) air pressure necessary for expiration to the lower (negative) air pressure necessary for inspiration.

If a speaker moves his larynx into the phonation position during an expiration and does nothing to change the tensions of the various laryngeal muscles, then the fundamental frequency of phonation will be determined by the transglottal air pressure drop (Lieberman, 1967; Atkinson, 1973; Collier, 1975). Müller (1848) first noted that the rate at which the vocal cords open and close, which determines the fundamental frequency of phonation, is a function of the air pressure differential across the vocal cords. If a speaker maintains a relatively unobstructed supralaryngeal airway and keeps his larynx in a fixed phonation position, then the fundamental frequency will be determined by the pulmonary air pressure. These conditions are met in the cries of newborn humans (Truby, Bosma and Lind, 1965); the supralaryngeal vocal tract's configuration is maintained throughout the cry and phonation occurs until the very end of the breath-group. The fundamental frequency at the end of the breath-group in these cries always falls. The fundamental frequency must fall because, in the absence of increased activity of the laryngeal muscles, the pulmonary air pressure goes from a positive to a negative value at the end of the breath-group. The transition in pulmonary air pressure is a consequence of the act of breathing. The form of the normal breath-group is a condition of minimum departure from the constraints of vegetative breathing. A speaker has to generate a negative air pressure in the lungs in order to inspire air. If the muscles that control the larynx simply "set" the proper medial compression and neutral position for phonation, then f_0 will be a function of the transglottal air pressure drop.

There can be various f_0 variations throughout the breath-group. The one certain aspect of the breath-group will be *the fall in f_0 at the breath-group's end*. The pulmonary air pressure must rapidly fall at the end of the expiration from

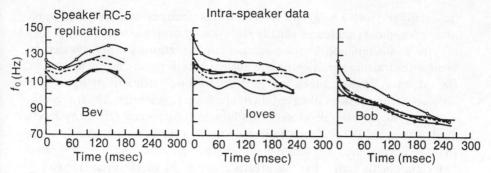

Figure 8.17. Fundamental frequency contours derived from one speaker's production of five tokens of the sentence Bev loves Bob. *Note that the speaker does not produce the same absolute fundamental frequency contour for each token. Note that the greatest consistency occurs at the end of the sentence where the fundamental frequency falls. (After Atkinson, 1973.)*

the positive pressure of the nonterminal part of the breath-group to the negative pressure of inspiration. The f_0 contour therefore must fall *unless* the speaker executes compensating maneuvers with his laryngeal muscles. In the absence of compensating maneuvers, f_0 must fall. If the speaker anticipates the beginning of inspiration and opens his larynx towards the end of the breath-group, the f_0 contour will fall still faster. The vibrating mass of the vocal cords will increase, causing f_0 to fall faster; the aerodynamic and aerostatic forces will fall as the phonation neutral position becomes more open. In short, everything that can occur to hasten the start of inspiration will cause f_0 to fall. This is the basis of the normal or unmarked breath-group. The plots reproduced from Atkinson (1973) in Figure 8.17 show the variations in f_0 traces of the same person repeating the simple sentence *Bev loves Bob*. Note the variations in the f_0 contours except at the end of the breath-group. Note also the regularity in the duration of each syllable. Many of the perceptual interpretations of prosody that are ascribed to f_0 variations may, in fact, reflect variations in the durations of segments. In particular, the duration of the last syllable of the breath-group is lengthened and furnishes a perceptually salient cue for the end of the breath-group (Klatt, 1976). The perceptually based phonetic transcriptions of linguists often conflate an f_0 fall with an increase in the duration of the terminal syllable of a breath-group (Lieberman, 1965). Systematic changes in duration also occur at phrase boundaries (Klatt, 1976; Cooper and Cooper, 1980).

Although the "easiest" or "most natural" way of producing a breath-group appears to be the state of minimal control that results in a terminal falling f_0 contour, some speakers produce terminal falling f_0 contours by other means (Lieberman, 1967; Ohala, 1970). The "ordinary" sentences of certain speakers habitually end with a rising or a level f_0. If these speakers are using a language in which ordinary sentences usually end with a normal $-$*breath-group*, they may be misunderstood because linguistic information is often signaled by using a contrasting variation on the normal breath-group. Many languages, for example, English, make use of a contrasting intonational signal that involves a rising or not-falling terminal f_0 contour (Lieberman, 1967) as well as a slightly higher overall average fundamental frequency (Hadding-Koch, 1961; Atkinson, 1973). The notation $-$*breath-group* (which implicitly states that the normal breath-group is the unmarked pattern) and $+$*breath-group* (which implicitly states that this breath-group is the marked pattern) can be used to differentiate these patterns. In English, yes–no questions are typically produced with a $+$*breath-group* (Lieberman, 1967).

The $+$*breath-group* that is used in normal yes–no questions in English appears to be structured by its acoustic contrast with the $-$*breath-group*. Whereas the f_0 contour may vary throughout the $-$*breath-group's* nonterminal portion, it falls at the end of the breath-group. In the $+$*breath-group*, f_0 does *not* fall at the end. (In a sense the $+$*breath-group* is structured by physiological constraints $-$ because it is in opposition to the $-$*breath-group*, which is clearly structured by the constraints of respiration, being a state of minimum departure from the vegetative function of respiration.) The manner in which a speaker produces a $+$*breath-group* appears to be quite complex. A number of studies (cf. Chapter 6) have shown that muscles like the sternohyoid, which is one of the muscles that adjusts the hyoid bone, which supports the larynx, is often active when f_0 variations occur during phonation. It is possible that this muscle and the muscles that set the phonation neutral position of the larynx, may act to switch the larynx from the lower chest register that is used for a $-$*breath-group* to a high chest register during a $+$*breath-group*. The data available at this moment are still rather fragmentary and limited to a few speakers of English, Japanese and Swedish.

The state of our understanding of the physiological and perceptual bases of the breath-group is not very different from that of most of the hypothetical phonetic features that we have discussed. We have some good data and several reasonable hypotheses. Many of the studies of the underlying physiology of the prosodic features have derived data that indicate that variations in pulmonary air pressure have only a small effect on the fundamental frequency of phonation (Ohala, 1970; Vanderslice and Ladefoged, 1972). Vanderslice and Ladefoged (1972) also interpret the intonation pattern that corresponds to the normal breath-group as a unified entity. They use the term *cadence* to describe the total pattern that segments a sentence.

A number of recent studies (Maeda, 1976; Pierrehumbert, 1979; Cooper and Sorenson, 1981) take a position opposite to that of the breath-group theory.

202

These studies claim that a gradual fall in f_0 throughout a sentence is a linguistic universal and that this gradual fall – the "declination" – is the acoustic cue that listeners use to segment the flow of speech into sentences. These studies suggest that the "declination line," used to characterize the sentence-level aspects of f_0, furnishes a psychologically real baseline for the perception of segmental stress (Pierrehumbert, 1979). However, it is not clear that declination is universal. Analyses of the intonation of American English, British English and Mandarin Chinese (Lieberman, Landahl and Ryalls, 1982; Tseng, 1981; Umeda, 1982; Lieberman *et al.*, 1985; Remez, Rubin and Nygaard, 1986) have failed to show declination for many utterances in both read and spontaneous speech. It is hoped that further research will resolve this issue.

The perceptual value of the acoustic phenomena that occur at the end of a breath-group (or cadence pattern) is also still not fully understood. Changes in the tempo of speech, for example, usually appear to typify the end of a breath-group. The duration of segments becomes longer at the breath-group's end. The glottal spectrum also typically loses energy in higher harmonics of the fundamental during the last few glottal periods. All of these events may serve as acoustic cues signalling the end of a breath-group. It is not certain that they actually have much importance, because appropriate perceptual experiments have yet to be performed. It is often possible to isolate acoustic phenomena that are *not* important to human listeners. Irregularities in the fundamental frequency, for example, commonly occur at the start and end of the phonation but human listeners are not aware of either the presence or the absence of these "perturbations" (Lieberman and Michaels, 1963).

Linguistic universals and biological structuring

The reader may have noted an apparent inconsistency in the discussion of the breath-group. We first made a strong case for the "naturalness" of the *– breath-group*. We then stated that speakers sometimes do not make use of this pattern of activity and instead produce sounds that have contrasting acoustic properties. The situation would be simple if all languages, and all speakers, behaved like our hypothetical "normal" speaker of English. Most sentences would be produced using the unmarked *– breath-group* by means of the pattern of least muscular control that we have discussed. The more costly, "marked" *+ breath-group* would be reserved for fewer sentences. Unfortunately, some speakers of English produce *– breath-group* by means of "odd" patterns of articulatory activity that involve more articulatory control than they could have used (Lieberman, 1967). Worse still is the fact that some languages appear to use *+ breath-group* patterns for most of their sentences. If the biological constraints *determined* the sound pattern of all human languages, then we should expect to find a universal invariant pattern.

The answer is that the biological constraints *structure* the possible forms of human language although they *do not determine the form* of language. The relation that holds between certain biological constraints and the possible form of the sound pattern may be very strong without being entirely deterministic. The biological mechanisms that underlie *voicing*, for example, appear to be as controlling as the biological factors that underlie upright bipedal posture in humans. However, it is possible to devise a human language in which all sounds are + *voiced*. The key to understanding the properties of human speech is that of determining the biological mechanisms that structure possible phonetic features. We cannot isolate these mechanisms if we insist that the appropriate criterion is that the particular mechanism is always manifested. For example, the biological mechanisms that structure human bipedal posture and locomotion are present in all normal humans. We would not dismiss the significance of these mechanisms if we found a "crucial" case of a normal human being who, like Tom Scott, the assistant to the villainous Quilp in Dickens' *Old Curiosity Shop*, habitually walked upright on his hands. There is no reason why a structuring principle must be universally manifested. Various groups of people for various peculiar reasons might not make use of some sounds, e.g. bilabials, although they were highly valued and although most languages use these sounds (Jakobson, 1968).

Exercises

1. Imagine that you are evaluating a proposal for a research grant. You have to decide whether the proposed project is scientifically sound. The proposal involves an elaborate X-ray machine that will track the position of a speaker's tongue while he talks. The speaker's lips and larynx must be shielded in order to minimize exposure to radiation so no information on the activity of the lips or the position of the larynx will be available. The study intends to derive new information on vowel production. Present a critique of the proposed experiment.

2. What are the acoustic properties of a "quantal" sound?

3. How does the shape of the human tongue and muscles like the styloglossus (cf. Chapter 6) facilitate the production of quantal vowels?

4. Compare and contrast the motor theory of speech with the theory of acoustic invariance. In what ways are they similar, and dissimilar?

9

Some current topics in speech research

The evolution of human speech

As we have noted throughout this book, human speech appears to involve a number of innate, i.e. genetically transmitted, anatomical and neural mechanisms. The plurality of these mechanisms is consistent with the mosaic nature of evolution (Mayr, 1982), which basically states that living organisms are put together in genetically transmitted "bits and pieces." Some of these mechanisms appear to be species-specific. Other aspects of human language, which are beyond the scope of this book, like rule-governed syntax, may also involve species-specific neural mechanisms. These species-specific anatomical and neural mechanisms probably evolved to enhance human linguistic ability. As we noted in Chapter 7, human speech allows us to transmit phonetic "segments" at a rate of up to 25 segments per second. In contrast, it is impossible to identify other nonspeech data at rates that exceed 7–9 items per second. A short two second long sentence can contain about 50 sound segments. The previous sentence, for example, which consists of approximately 50 phonetic segments, can be uttered in two seconds. If this sentence had to be transmitted at the rate of nonspeech, it would take so long that a human listener would forget the beginning of the sentence before hearing its end. The high data transmission rate of human speech thus is an integral part of human linguistic ability that allows complex thoughts to be transmitted within the constraints of short-term memory.

The process by which this high transmission rate is achieved involves the generation of formant frequency patterns and rapid temporal and spectral cues by the species-specific human supralaryngeal airway and its associated neural control mechanism. The human supralaryngeal airway differs from that of any other adult mammal (Negus, 1949). Figure 9.1 shows the typical nonhuman airway of a chimpanzee in which the tongue is positioned entirely within the oral cavity where it forms the lower margin. The midsagittal view shows the airway as it would appear if the animal were sectioned on its midline from front to back. The position of the long, relatively thin tongue reflects the high position of the larynx. The larynx locks into the nasopharynx during respiration, providing a pathway for air from the nose to the lungs that is isolated from liquid that may be in the animal's mouth. Nonhuman mammals

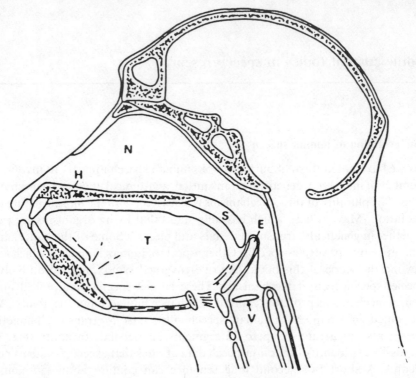

Figure 9.1. Midsagittal view of the head of an adult chimpanzee; N, nasal cavity; H, hard palate; S, soft palate; E, epiglottis; T, tongue; V, vocal cords of larynx. (Adapted from Laitman and Heimbuch, 1982.) From Lieberman, 1984.

retain this morphology throughout their lives, as do human infants until aged three months. Given this morphology, nonhuman mammals and young infants can simultaneously breathe and drink (Laitman, Crelin and Conlogue, 1977). The ingested fluid moves to either side of the raised larynx which resembles a raised periscope protruding through the oral cavity, connecting the lungs with the nose. Figure 9.2 shows the human configuration. The larynx has lowered into the neck. The tongue's contour in the midsagittal plane is round; it forms the anterior (forward) margin of the pharynx as well as the lower margin of the oral cavity. Air, liquids and solid food make use of the common pharyngeal pathway. Humans thus are more liable to die when they eat because food can fall into the larynx obstructing the pathway into the lungs. The peculiar deficiencies of the human supralaryngeal vocal tract for swallowing have long been noted. Darwin (1859, p.191) for example, noted "the strange fact that every particle of food and drink which we swallow has to pass over the orifice of the trachea, with some risk of falling into the lungs."

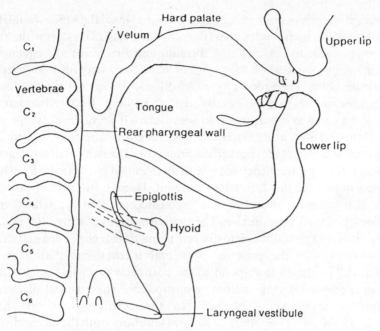

Figure 9.2. Midsagittal view of the adult human supralaryngeal vocal tract. From Lieberman, 1984.

During ontogenetic development, the human palate moves back with respect to the bottom, i.e. the base, of the skull (Crelin, 1969). The base of the human adult skull is restructured compared to all other mammals to achieve this supralaryngeal airway. The adult human configuration is less efficient for chewing because the length of the palate (the roof of the mouth) and mandible (lower jaw) have been reduced. The reduced length of the palate and mandible also crowd our teeth presenting the possibility of infection due to impaction – a potentially fatal condition until the advent of modern dentistry. These vegetative deficiencies are, however, offset by the increased phonetic range of the human supralaryngeal airway. The round human tongue moving in the right-angle space defined by the palate and spinal column can generate formant frequency patterns like those that define vowels like [i], [u], and [a] and consonants like [k] and [g] (Lieberman and Crelin, 1971; Lieberman, 1973, 1975, 1984). As we noted in Chapter 8, these quantal sounds of human speech appear to be better suited for vocal communication than other sounds.

As we have noted earlier, the perception of human speech is a complex process that appears to involve a number of innate, genetically transmitted neural mechanisms. Specialized neural mechanisms operate at different stages in a "speech mode" of perception in which human listeners appear to apply

207

different strategies or mechanisms to an acoustic signal than they would if they thought it was a nonspeech signal (Remez *et al.*, 1981). To start with, human listeners are able to "extract" the formant and fundamental frequencies of speech signals, even when these signals have been degraded by telephone circuits or noise. The process by which human beings extract the formant frequencies appears to involve the listener's "knowing" the filtering character-istics of the supralaryngeal airway at some internal neural level of representa-tion (Halle and Stevens, 1959). Human listeners must also form an estimate of the probable length of the speaker's supralaryngeal airway in order to assign a particular formant frequency pattern to an intended phonetic target. Human listeners must take this factor into account. Human listeners in the speech mode also integrate an ensemble of acoustic cues that are related by the physiology of speech production. They assign patterns of formant frequencies and short-term spectral cues into discrete phonetic categories in a manner that is consistent with the presence of neural mechanisms that have been "matched," i.e. tuned to respond to the particular acoustic signals that the human speech-producing anatomy can produce. These neural mechanisms appear to have been "matched" to the constraints of the human supralaryngeal airway by means of natural selection. Both the motor theory of speech perception (Chapter 7) and the phonetic theory involving invariant acoustic properties (Chapter 8) involve at some neural level perceptual mechanisms that are adapted to process sounds that can be produced by the species-specific human supralaryngeal vocal tract. These perceptual mechan-isms also may involve more general auditory processes. These specialized speech detectors appear to be homologues of simpler ones that have been identified using electrophysiological and behavioral techniques in other species.

The production of human speech likewise involves species-specific neural mechanisms. Broca first identified the area of the brain in which the motor programs that underlie the production of human speech are stored. The articulatory maneuvers that underlie the production of human speech appear to be the most complex that human beings attain. Normal children are not up to adult criteria until aged ten years (Watkin and From, 1984). Human speakers are able to execute complex coordinated articulatory maneuvers involving the tongue, lips, velum, larynx and lungs that are directed towards linguistic goals, e.g. producing a particular formant frequency pattern. Pongids who lack Broca's area likewise cannot be taught to control their supralaryngeal airways to produce any human speech sounds. Although the nonhuman pongid airway inherently cannot produce all of the sounds of human speech, it could produce a subset of human speech sounds. Nonhuman primates lacking Broca's area are unable to produce even these sounds. The homologue of Broca's area in nonhuman primates may be the lateral precentral cortex which is involved in the regulation of oro-facial gestures for communication (Deacon, 1985). Speech communication may be the selective force for the evolution of Broca's area and the elaboration of oro-facial articulation.

The evolution of the human supralaryngeal airway and matching perceptual mechanisms is probably similar in kind to the match between anatomy and auditory perception that has been demonstrated in other species such as crickets, frogs and monkeys. Human speech makes use of anatomical structures and neural perceptual mechanisms that also occur in other species, e.g. the larynx is similar for all apes, rodents and primates, and chinchillas possess the auditory mechanisms for the perception of certain linguistic cues (voice-onset time) (Kuhl and Miller, 1974, 1975; Kuhl, 1981). However, the anatomy and neural control mechanisms that are necessary for the production of complex formant frequency patterns appear to have evolved comparatively recently, in the last 1.4 million years. Comparative and fossil studies indicate that the human supralaryngeal vocal tract may have started to evolve in hominid populations like that of the *Homo habilis* KNM-ER 3733 fossil (Lieberman, 1984, 1985). However, some more recent hominids like classic Neanderthal retained the nonhuman supralaryngeal vocal tract; other hominids contemporary with Neanderthal had human supralaryngeal airways. The vegetative deficiencies of the human supralaryngeal airway are outweighed only by the adaptive value of rapid human speech. In the absence of the matching neural mechanisms, it would not be possible to produce the complex articulatory maneuvers that are necessary for speech production, nor would it be possible to perceptually decode the speech signal.

Ontogenetic development of speech

It is becoming apparent that the development of speech starts early in the first year of life. As we discussed in Chapter 7, infants as young as several days old display categorical-like perception for the sounds of speech. In particular, they discriminate the sounds of speech in a manner similar to adults. The discrimination experiment with infants makes use of an ingenious technique in which infants are trained to suck a rubber nipple when they hear "new" sounds (Eimas *et al.*, 1971; Cutting and Eimas, 1975). The infant is given a hand-held nipple to suck on. Instead of transferring nutrients, the nipple contains a pressure transducer which records the force and the rate at which the infant sucks. These signals are recorded on a polygraph and a digital recording. Contingent on the sucking response is the presentation of an auditory stimulus. The rate at which stimuli are presented to the infant can be made proportional to the rate at which the infant sucks. The infant soon learns that more presentations of a stimuli will occur if he sucks more often. What occurs is that infants want more presentations of sounds that they perceive to be different from the sound that they heard before. If the same stimulus is presented many times to an infant, the infant's sucking rate will decrease as he becomes satiated with the sound. If a sound that the infant hears as different is presented, the infant will become interested again and suck more rapidly. The infant's satiation and curiosity make this experiment a discrimination test. The experimenter presents a signal until the infant is satiated. The experimenter then can present a different acoustic signal. If the infant can perceive that the new sound is different, the sucking rate increases abruptly. If the infant is not able to discriminate the new acoustic signal from the "old" acoustic signal, he remains satiated and does not increase his sucking rate. The results of these experiments with infants ranging in age from several days to four months is extremely important because they show that the discrimination boundaries of infants and adults appear to be similar for the sounds of human speech. These results are, of course, consistent with a theory that involves innately determined neural property detectors. Kuhl (1979a) in her review of the data on speech perception in infants shows that they can discriminate virtually all the sound contrasts that enter into English as well as the fundamental frequency patterns that are used for phonemic tones in many other languages.

Interestingly, infants show categorical-like discrimination even for sounds that may not occur in their language. For example, in Hindi there is a distinction between retroflex stops (produced by curling the tongue back and placing it posterior to the alveolar ridge) and dental stops, as well as a distinction between voiced and voiceless aspirated stops. In contrast, English has neither contrast, and alveolar stops rather than dental stops are found. Werker and her colleagues (Werker *et al.*, 1981) attempted to determine whether seven-month-old infants of English-speaking parents could discriminate these (non-English) Hindi speech contrasts. Results showed that they could, despite having had no exposure to these speech sounds. Moreover, she found that if infants were not exposed to such speech sounds, there was a decline in their ability to discriminate such phonetic distinctions. Evidence for this decline was seen by the end of the first year of life (Werker and Tees, 1984).

These results clearly indicate that infants are born with a predisposition to perceive the sounds of language, and while experience with language is necessary for "tuning" the particular language system being acquired, the basic perceptual mechanisms for speech seem to be in place at birth. However, Werker's findings also show that language exposure is critical for maintaining these discrimination abilities.

Kuhl (Kuhl, 1979a, 1979b, 1980, 1986; Kuhl and Miller, 1982) in a series of ingenious studies has also shown that six-month-old infants are able to not only discriminate speech stimuli, but also to categorize them. Using a head-turning reinforcement procedure, she has demonstrated that infants show *perceptual equivalence* for vowels when they are produced by different talkers and when the vowels vary in fundamental frequency. Thus, they treat all tokens of [a] as the same or as *perceptually equivalent*, and all tokens of [i] as *perceptually equivalent*, despite variations in speaker and fundamental frequency. Similar findings have been shown for the perception of the nasal consonants [m] and [n] in different vowel environments (Hillenbrand, 1984).

The development of speech production seems to be much slower than that of speech perception. Though the start of the process of speech production is evident in the second month of life (Sandner, 1981; Lieberman, 1984), children usually start to talk in the second year of life. They are able to produce many basic acoustic cues that specify the speech sounds of their native language, e.g. vowel formant frequency patterns (Lieberman, 1980), consonantal onset cues for place of articulation (Chapin, Tseng and Lieberman, 1982), and voice-onset time (Port and Preston, 1972). However, their speech production ability only approximates the adult model (Clark and Clark, 1977; Landahl, 1982; Mack and Lieberman, 1985). Some sounds like [w], [r], and [l] present special problems (Kuehn and Tomblin, 1977). The development of adult-like muscular coordination is a long process. Figure 9.3, for example, shows the gradual development of the formant frequency pattern for the vowels of American English in an infant from age 16 to 62 weeks (Lieberman, 1980). Note that the vowel space gradually begins to approximate the adult model (c.f. Figures 8.8 and 8.9).

Watkin and Fromm (1984) show that the process is not complete at age ten years for even simple aspects of speech articulation like the lip movements that are necessary for the production of the vowels of English. Even voice-onset time is not fully stable until the child is about eight-years-old (Port and Preston, 1972). As we noted earlier (Chapters 6, 7 and 8), the articulatory gestures that underlie the production of speech are encoded, complex, and goal-directed. It is becoming evident that phenomena like coarticulation involve a speaker's somehow "learning" the patterns that are appropriate to his language. Lubker and Gay (1982), for example, show that native speakers of Swedish and American English differ as to how they move their lips in the "anticipatory" coarticulation of the vowel [u]. Adult speakers round their lips as they produce the sound [t] in the environment [tu] in anticipation of the vowel [u]; in contrast they do not round their lips when they produce the syllable [ti]. Speakers of English differ from speakers of Swedish in that they do not round their lips until 100 milliseconds before the start of the [u]. Some speakers of Swedish start rounding their lips 300 milliseconds before the [u].

211

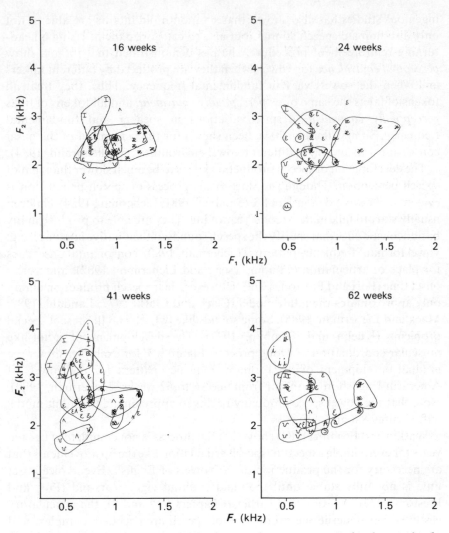

Figure 9.3. Gradual development of the formant frequency pattern for the vowels of American English in an infant from age 16 to 62 weeks.

The different patterns of anticipatory coarticulation are obviously learned as children acquire their native language, but the ontogenetic pattern of acquisition of these subtle distinctions is at present unclear. We likewise do not know very much about the acquisition of the factors that determine whether one has a "native" accent (Flege, 1984; Mack, 1983). Many theories of language acquisition claim that a "critical period" or "critical periods" exist that set limits on the ability of a person to acquire various aspects of linguistic

212

ability (Lenneberg, 1967; Lieberman, 1984). The degree to which the acquisition of speech reflects a special "language acquisition device," the maturation of neural structures, or associative learning is not clear. A wide range of opinion has been expressed, ranging from theories that stress language-specific mechanisms (Pinker, 1984) to general motor and cognitive development (Piaget, 1980; Snow, 1977).

Speech pathologies

The effects of malformations of the supralaryngeal vocal tract have long been noted. The effects of cleft palate, for example, have been studied in great detail (Folkins, 1985). Recent studies have examined the effects of other physical anomalies. Apert and Cruzon's syndromes are craniofacial developmental anomalies that result in congenitally anomalous supralaryngeal vocal tracts. The palate is positioned in a posterior position relative to its normal orientation with respect to the face and the pharynx is constricted. Landahl and Gould (1986) use computer models based on radiographic data to show that the phonetic output of subjects having these syndromes is limited by their supralaryngeal vocal tracts. The subjects attempt to model their vowels on normal speech, but their vocal tracts cannot produce the formant frequency range of normal speech. Psychoacoustic tests of their productions yield a 30 percent error rate for computer-excised vowels. Acoustic analysis of their speech shows that they are unable to produce the quantal vowels [i] and [u].

Figure 9.4 shows the results of a computer modeling of an Apert's subject. The loops of the Peterson and Barney (1952) study are shown on the F_1 and F_2 formant frequency plot. The vowel symbols clustered towards the center of these loops represent the formant frequency patterns that the Apert's supralaryngeal vocal tract can produce when the experimenters attempted to perturb it towards the best approximation of a normal vocal tract's configuration for each vowel. Note the absence of [i]'s or [u]'s. These data indicate that the normal supralaryngeal vocal tract is optimized to achieve a maximum phonetic output. Apert's syndrome in a sense is the result of the palate continuing to move back on the base of the skull past its "normal" position during ontogenetic development. These data support the hypothesis that an enhanced phonetic output was the primary selective force in the restructuring of the human supralaryngeal vocal tract in the last 100 to 250 thousand years. The "normal" configuration of the human supralaryngeal vocal tract yields the maximum formant frequency range. Configurations in which the palate is anterior (Lieberman, Crelin and Klatt, 1972) or posterior (Landahl and Gould, 1986) yield a reduced range of formant frequency patterns and hence a reduced phonetic inventory.

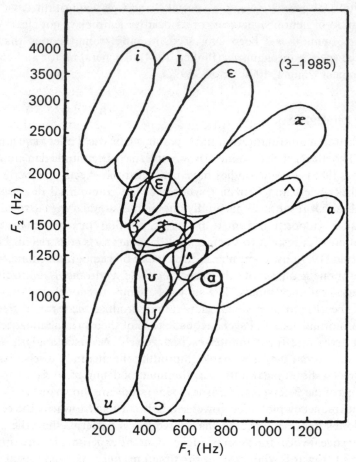

Figure 9.4. Computer modeling of vowel production in an Apert's subject.

Aphasia

An area of research that has provided a window into the organization of speech and language in the brain is *aphasia*. Aphasia is, by definition, a speech-language disorder resulting from neurological damage. The study of aphasia may be considered an "experiment in nature." This is because neurological damage may occur in different sites of the brain, and researchers can then explore what types of disorders arise from such damage. Of course, one must wait for such experiments to occur, since ethically the researcher cannot take normal subjects and damage certain portions of their brain to "see what would happen." However, nature does provide much of this information. People have strokes, they have neurological diseases, and they have all types of accidents and traumas. The resulting effects of brain damage on their normal abilities can then be explored.

For most right-handed adults, damage to certain areas of the left hemisphere produce some types of speech-language disturbance, whereas damage to the right hemisphere rarely affects speech-language processing *per se*. Moreover, different types of language disturbances are found depending upon the location of the lesion in the left hemisphere. For example, patients with Broca's aphasia usually have brain damage in the anterior portions of the left hemisphere. While their language comprehension is fairly good, the speech output of Broca's aphasics is usually slow and laboured. Articulation and speech melody or prosody are usually impaired, as is grammatical structure. In contrast, Wernicke's aphasics, with damage to the posterior portions of the left hemisphere, have fluent, well-articulated speech which seems to be relatively intact grammatically. Nevertheless, their speech output is often meaningless and empty of content. In addition, Wernicke's aphasics find it difficult to understand spoken language.

Nearly all aphasic patients display some impairments in both speech production and speech perception. What is important to understand is what the nature of these production and perception impairments might be. Such understanding will not only provide important clues about the organization of speech in the brain and its relation to language, but it may also help speech pathologists devise effective rehabilitation programs.

Investigations of the speech production of aphasic patients have shown some important differences between Broca's and Wernicke's aphasics. These studies have undertaken acoustic analyses of the production of certain phonetic attributes of speech. By exploring the acoustic characteristics of these attributes and comparing them to the productions of normal subjects, they can infer the nature and underlying basis of the disorder.

As we discussed earlier in Chapter 8, most languages of the world contrast voiced and voiceless consonants by varying *voicing onset*. In the production of stop consonants, *voicing onset* or *voice-onset time* (VOT) is the timing relation between the release of a stop consonant and the onset of glottal excitation. In a language like English, voiced consonants are either prevoiced, i.e. glottal excitation begins prior to the release of the stop consonant, or they have a short-lag VOT, i.e. the glottal excitation begins some 5–15 milliseconds after the release of the stop. In contrast, voiceless stops have a long-lag VOT, i.e. glottal excitation begins some 30 milliseconds or more after the release of the

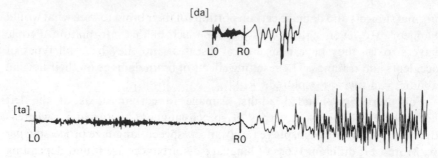

Figure 9.5. Waveform of a portion of a syllable beginning with a voiced and voiceless stop consonant. The positions of the cursors indicate the landmarks for measurement of VOT.

stop closure. Figure 9.5 shows a waveform of a portion of a syllable beginning with a voiced and voiceless stop consonant. The left cursor indicates the onset of the burst (the release of the stop closure) and the right cursor indicates the onset of glottal excitation (the quasi-periodic portion of the waveform). VOT is the time in milliseconds between these two points in time.

Experiments with normal subjects have shown that if they are asked to produce a series of words in isolation, each beginning with a voiced stop consonant, e.g. [d] in *dot*, or a voiceless stop consonant, e.g. [t] in *top*, and the VOT of each utterance is measured and then plotted, the distribution of voiced and voiceless responses falls into two clear-cut categories, with virtually no overlap between the two categories (Lisker and Abramson, 1964). The top panel of Figure 9.6 shows such a distribution. As the bottom panel of the figure shows, Wernicke's aphasics also produce two distinct categories of voiced and voiceless stops. In contrast, Broca's aphasics show a different pattern of VOT responses. In particular, as shown in the middle panel of Figure 9.6, there is not only overlap in VOT in the production of voiced and voiceless stop consonants, but in addition, VOT values fall in the range of 20–40 milliseconds, a range *between* the two categories of VOT for normal subjects. Thus, Broca's aphasics seem to be unable to control the timing between the release of a stop consonant and the onset of voicing (Blumstein *et al.*, 1977b, 1980; Freeman, Sands and Harris, 1978; Itoh *et al.*, 1982; Shewan, Leeper and Booth, 1984; Tuller, 1984). This pattern of performance is found not only in English and Japanese, languages which have two categories of voicing, but also in Thai, a language which has a three-category distinction for voicing – prevoicing, short-lag and long-lag VOT (Gandour and Dardarananda, 1984; cf. Chapter 8, pp. 196 ff).

That Broca's aphasics display a timing deficit in speech production,

216

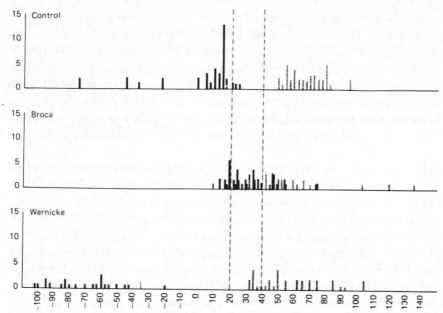

Figure 9.6. The distribution of VOT productions for the alveolar stop consonants for a normal control, a Broca's aphasic, and a Wernicke's aphasic. From S.E. Blumstein, Neurolinguistics: Language-brain relationships. In S.B. Filskov and T.J. Boll (eds.), Handbook of Clinical Neuropsychology. Reprinted by permission of John Wiley & Sons, Inc. Copyright © 1981.

particularly when it involves the timing of two independent articulators, is supported by an additional set of findings involving the production of nasal consonants. To produce a nasal consonant as [m] or [n], it is necessary to open the velum while releasing the closure in the oral cavity. Broca's aphasics also have difficulty in timing the release of the oral closure and the opening of the velum in the production of nasal consonants (Itoh, Sasanuma and Ushijima, 1979).

Although a timing disorder is clearly implicated in the speech production of Broca's aphasics, acoustic analyses of the spectral characteristics of stop consonants suggest that these patients seem to be able to get their vocal tract into the appropriate configuration for place of articulation in stop consonants (Shinn and Blumstein, 1983), and they seem to be able to produce the appropriate formant frequencies for vowels (Ryalls, 1986). Moreover, these patients also show relatively normal coarticulation effects in the transitions between consonants and vowels (Katz, 1986), although these effects may be somewhat delayed in time (Kent and Rosenbek, 1983; Ziegler and Von Cramon, 1985).

While Broca's and Wernicke's aphasics seem to differ with respect to

217

articulatory timing, both types of patients produce many similar types of speech errors. These errors include: phoneme substitution errors in which one sound is substituted for another, e.g. *teams* → [kimz]; simplification errors in which a sound or syllable is deleted, e.g. *green* → [gin]; addition errors in which an extra sound or syllable is added, e.g. *see* → [sti]; and environment errors in which a particular sound error that occurs can be accounted for by the influence of the surrounding phonetic environment, e.g. *roast beef* → [rof bif]. Note that the final consonant cluster of the word *roast* is *assimilated* to the final [f] of *beef* (Blumstein, 1973).

It is worth noting that analyses of the phoneme substitution errors of aphasics are consistent with the view that sound segments are comprised of phonetic features. As we discussed in Chapter 8, many linguists and speech researchers have suggested that sound segments are comprised of a bundle of phonetic features. When patients substitute one sound segment for another, the substituted sound is usually different by one phonetic feature from that of the attempted or target sound. For example, patients may make voicing errors, *doll* → [tal], place errors, e.g. *teams* → [kimz], but they rarely make errors involving both voicing and place errors in the same sound substitution, e.g. *doll* → *[kal]. Nearly all aphasics show this same pattern of errors.

Speech production impairments are not the only type of speech deficit found in aphasic patients. Many aphasics also show speech perception impairments. They often have difficulty in discriminating words or nonsense syllables which contrast by a single phonetic feature, e.g. *bait* vs. *date* or [beip] vs. [deip] (Blumstein *et al.*, 1977a; Jauhianen and Nuutila, 1977; Miceli *et al.*, 1978; Miceli *et al.*, 1980; Baker, Blumstein and Goodglass, 1981). The testing procedures are quite simple and straightforward. The patient is presented via a tape recording with pairs of words or nonsense syllables, such as *bait–date* or *bait–bait*. On each trial, he is asked to press a key marked YES if the two stimuli are the same, and NO if the two stimuli are different. In this way, the patient need only press a button. He does not have to speak which may be very difficult. Results of such discrimination tests have shown that aphasic patients, regardless of type of aphasia, have more difficulty discriminating words or nonsense syllables which contrast by a single phonetic feature than by more than one feature, and they have particular difficulty when that contrast is for place of articulation.

If aphasic patients have difficulty discriminating stimuli contrasting in voicing or place of articulation, perhaps they will not show categorical perception of the sounds of speech. As we discussed in Chapter 7, adult listeners show categorical perception of speech in that they are able to discriminate between sounds reliably *only* when the pair of sounds they are discriminating between lie across a category boundary. Moreover, infants as young as a few days old also show categorical-like discrimination functions. How would aphasics perform on such tasks?

Studies exploring categorical perception in aphasics have focused on two phonetic dimensions – voicing (Basso, Casati and Vignolo, 1977; Blumstein *et al.*, 1977b; Gandour and Dardarananda, 1982) and place of articulation (Blumstein *et al.*, 1984). The stimuli used in these studies were computer-generated. One series varied in VOT to explore the voiced–voiceless dimension. The other series explored the dimension of place of articulation. The stimuli varied in the frequency of the formant transitions apropriate for the syllables [ba], [da] and [ga], and in the presence or absence of a burst preceding the transitions. Aphasic subjects were asked to perform two tasks. The first task was to identify the initial consonant by pointing to the appropriate written letter. The second task was to discriminate pairs of stimuli by pressing a button marked YES if the pair of stimuli were the same, and NO, if they were different. Three patterns of results emerged. One group of patients were able to perform the task like normal subjects and thus showed categorical perception. A second group found both tasks too difficult and could neither reliably identify nor discriminate the sounds. A third group, however, showed an interesting dissociation. They were unable to identify the sounds, but they were able to discriminate them. More importantly, as Figure 9.7 shows, they showed a categorical-like discrimination function. That is, they were only able to discriminate those stimuli which lay across a category boundary. More importantly, the shape of the obtained function and boundary values were similar to those found for subjects who could both identify and discriminate the stimuli. Thus, these aphasic patients showed discrimination boundaries that appear to be similar to those obtained for normal adults and for infants. These results underscore the stability of the categorical nature of speech.

Exercises

1. A brilliant surgeon devises a procedure for supralaryngeal vocal tract transplants. What would happen to the speech of an otherwise normal adult if the supralaryngeal vocal tract of an adult chimpanzee were exchanged with him? The person is an actor who wants to look authentic for a role in a movie about Australopithecines (human-like animals who lived between 3 and 1 million years ago).

   Would the chimpanzee be able to talk if he had the actor's human supralaryngeal vocal tract? Why?

2. What anatomical and neurological factors underlie the present form of human speech?

3. Children are said to acquire the intonation of their native language in the first year of life. How could you test this theory? In a paragraph or two present the procedures that you would use to test this hypothesis.

219

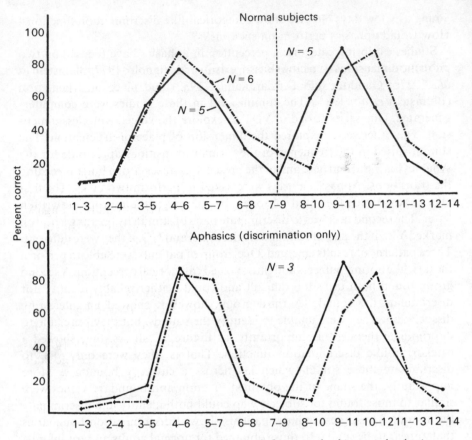

Figure 9.7. Discrimination of [ba da ga] stimuli for normal subjects and aphasics. The straight lines correspond to the burst plus transition stimuli and the dotted lines the transition only stimuli. The vertical line at stimulus pair 7–9 in the top and bottom panels indicate that the computed functions for the [b–d] discrimination pairs was based on a different number of subjects (N) than the [d–g] discrimination pairs. From Blumstein et al., 1984.

4. In what ways do the data from the acquisition of speech and pathology of speech provide different but critical insights into the nature of speech production and speech perception?

5. What differences are there between Broca's and Wernicke's aphasics in speech production? What do these results tell us about the neurological bases of speech production?

10

Acoustic correlates of speech sounds

We have discussed the sounds of speech in terms of articulatory and acoustic data and in terms of theoretical models of speech. In this last chapter, we present some of the acoustic correlates of various speech sounds of English. This review will not be a comprehensive study of the acoustic correlates of the sounds of human speech or even of the sounds of English, but it should be a useful starting point for more detailed study.

One of the challenges of speech research is to determine what aspects of the acoustic signal are relevant to the listener for perceiving the sounds of speech. As is apparent from the earlier discussions on the acoustics of speech, the speech signal is complex with temporal, durational and spectral variations. However, research has shown that listeners can perceive speech with a greatly "stripped down" version of the acoustic signal. In other words, only certain aspects of the acoustic signal seem to be relevant to the listener for perceiving the phonetic dimensions of speech. These relevant attributes for speech are called acoustic correlates or *acoustic cues*. Let us review some of the acoustic cues necessary for the perception of English speech sounds.

Vowels

The frequency positions of the first three formants are sufficient cues for listeners to identify the vowels of English. The formant frequency relations that specify the vowels of English are inherently relational rather than absolute since different-sized supralaryngeal vocal tracts will produce different absolute formant frequencies. Figure 10.1 shows the mean values of F_1, F_2, and F_3 of the vowels of American English spoken by adult males. Perhaps the best way to remember the formant frequency patterns is to start with the quantal vowels [i], [u] and [a]. The vowel [i] has the highest F_2 and F_3 of all English vowels. The convergence of F_2 and F_3 results in a well-defined high frequency peak in the spectrum of the vowel's transfer function. The vowel [i] also has a low F_1. The numbers entered on Figure 10.1 are the means derived from the Peterson and Barney (1952) analysis. The means of F_1, F_2 and F_3 of [i] are 270, 2290, and 3010 Hz respectively. Like [i], the vowel [u] also has a low F_1 at 300 Hz.

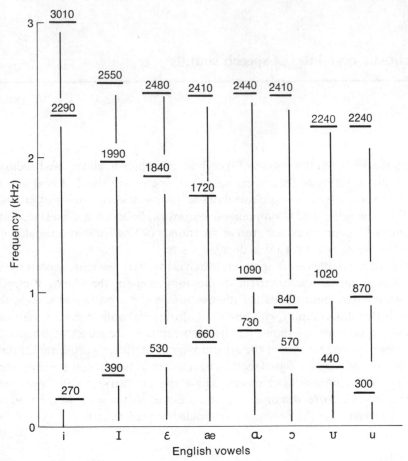

Figure 10.1. Mean values of formant frequencies for adult males of vowels of American English measured by Peterson and Barney (1952).

However, the F_2 of [u] is also low at 870 Hz. The vowel [ɑ] is specified by F_1 and F_2 converging towards each other at about 900 Hz in the middle region of the vowel space. Note that the "front" or "acute" vowels [i ɪ ɛ æ] have a high F_2 and the "back" or "grave" vowels [ɑ ɔ ʊ u] have a low F_2. Moreover, both [i] and [u], with a high tongue body position in the mouth, have a low F_1, whereas [ɑ], with a low tongue position, has a high F_1 (Nearey, 1978).

For the most part, vowels can be perceived correctly with only the first two formants (Delattre *et al.*, 1952; Fant, 1973). However, if only the first two formants are synthesized, then it is often necessary to use an "effective" second formant frequency (F'_2) which takes into account the shape of the spectrum that would have resulted if the higher formant frequencies were present. The formant frequencies used by Cooper *et al.* (1952) to synthesize [i] were, for example, 270 and 2700 Hz for F_1 and F_2, rather than 270 and 2290 Hz as shown in Figure 10.1.

Differences in vowel duration are also typical of the vowels in English, and duration does provide an additional cue for specifying vowel quality (cf. Miller, 1981, for a review). For example, Peterson and Lehiste (1960) measured the durations of vowels produced in words spoken in a sentence frame. Their results showed that the inherent duration of the vowels of English are different. For example, the vowels [ɪ] as in *hid*, [ɛ] as in *head*, and [ʊ] as in *hood* were the shortest, ranging in duration from 180 to 200 milliseconds. In contrast, the vowels [i] as in *heed*, [a] as in *hod* and [u] as in *who'd* ranged between 240 and 260 milliseconds, and [æ] as in *had* was 330 milliseconds. Many of the longer vowels of English are diphthongized (Peterson and Lehiste, 1960). The diphthongization generally consists of the formant frequency pattern going from that of one "pure" vowel to a second vowel or "semi-vowel," e.g. [ai] or [ay] in the word *bite* and [ɔi] or [ɔy] in the word *boy*. These durations are relative and depend on the rate of speech, the degree to which words are stressed, and the position of a word with respect to a phrase boundary or the end of a breath-group (Umeda, 1975; Klatt, 1976). Duration also changes as a function of context: when words are read in context, the average duration of vowels is reduced. Moreover, duration is more variable for spontaneous discourse than it is for read speech (Remez *et al.* 1986). Listeners seem to be sensitive to such duration changes, and often identify vowels as a function of their relative durations.

In English, vowels are usually produced with the velum raised against the back of the pharynx to shut off the nasal passages from the pharynx and oral tract. Vowels produced in this way are called *oral vowels*. However, speakers of English nasalize their vowels by opening the velum, particularly in those vowels preceding a nasal consonant, e.g. *can* → [kæn]. In some languages of the world, vowel nasalization is distinctive phonetically in that it is used to distinguish words of different meanings, e.g. in French *mot* [mo] meaning "word" is distinguished from *mon* [mõ] meaning "my." Research results on the perception of nasal and oral vowels in speakers of English (which does not have distinctive vowel nasalization) and other languages (which do have distinctive vowel nasalization) have shown that for all of the listeners, the primary acoustic cue for vowel nasalization is a reduction in the spectral prominence of the first formant. This is accomplished by either broadening the F_1 peak (making it wider in bandwidth) or creating an additional spectral peak nearby (Delattre, 1968; Hawkins and Stevens, 1985). The perceptual consequences of vowel nasalization are higher confusions when people are asked to identify them (Bond, 1976).

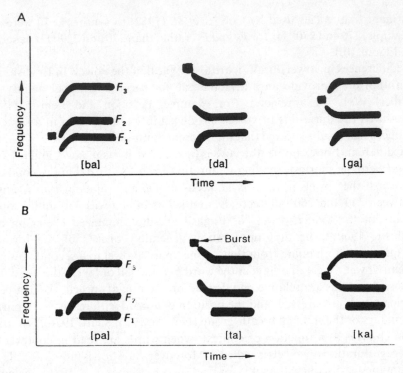

Figure 10.2. Formant transitions and bursts for the syllables [ba da ga pa ta ka].

Stop consonants

The stop consonants of English [p t k b d g] share the same manner of articulation in that they are produced with the rapid release of a complete closure in the vocal tract. There are several acoustic cues that contribute to the perception of a stop consonant. One is the release burst, and the other is the rate and duration of the formant transitions, particularly of the first formant (Liberman *et al.*, 1956; Keating and Blumstein, 1978). Both cues are the acoustic consequence of the rapid release of the stop closure. The duration of the burst is generally of the order of 5–15 milliseconds and that of the transitions is 20–40 milliseconds. Either cue alone will be sufficient for the listener to perceive a stop consonant.

The stop consonants [p b t d k g] vary in place of articulation – [p b] are labials, [t d] are alveolars and [k g] are velars. The acoustic cues to place of articulation in stop consonants include the spectrum of the burst release and formant transitions. In the top part of Figure 10.2, bursts and formant frequency patterns are shown for the consonant–vowel syllables [ba], [da] and [ga]. The steady-state formants correspond to the formant frequency values for the vowel [a]. Note that the second and third formants both rise from a lower frequency relative to the vowel steady-states for [ba], and are thus described as having *rising transitions*, and the burst is appended to the second formant transition. For [da], the second and third formants are *falling* relative to the vowel steady-state, and the burst excites F_3. And for [ga], the second and third formants diverge or "spread apart" from each other with F_2 falling and F_3 rising. The burst is juxtaposed to the F_2 and F_3 transitions. The frequency of the burst and the pattern of formant transitions give rise to the perception of different places of articulation. The actual frequencies at which the bursts occur and the formant transitions begin vary as a function of vowel context (Cooper *et al.*, 1952).

While the burst and transitions can be visually separated on a spectrogram, as is shown in the schematic drawing of Figure 10.2, it is not clear that the perceptual system separately extracts these cues in the perception of place of articulation in stop consonants. Rather, they may form a single *integrated* cue (Stevens and Blumstein, 1979). There is always a spectral continuity between the burst and formant transitions. That is, there is a continuity between the frequency spectrum of the burst and the frequency spectrum at the beginning of the formant transitions. Without this continuity, the perceptual performance for place of articulation is diminished (Dorman, Studdert-Kennedy and Raphael, 1977; Fischer-Jorgensen, 1972).

Among the stop consonants of English, [p t k] are voiceless and [b d g] are voiced. There are a multiple of acoustic cues distinguishing voiced and voiceless stops. One of the first that was systematically investigated was F_1 cutback. If formant frequency patterns for [ba da ga] as shown in Figure 10.2A are synthesized but with the F_1 transition portions eliminated, as shown in Figure 10.2B, then the consonants are perceived as voiceless, i.e. [p t k] (Cooper *et al.*, 1952). Moreover, when the F_2 and F_3 transitions are "excited" by noise rather than by voicing during the cutback interval, voicing responses are more consistently heard. The noise excitation in the transitions corresponds to noise generated at the glottis (Fant, 1960, p.19). Burst amplitude and aspiration amplitude also play a perceptual role, with greater values resulting in an increase in voiceless percepts (Repp, 1979). It is the combination of both F_1 cutback and aspiration which corresponds to the voice-onset time parameter which we discussed in Chapter 8.

Other acoustic cues also contribute to the voiced–voiceless distinction in stop consonants, particularly when the stop consonant appears in other phonetic environments such as between two vowels, e.g. [beikiŋ] *baking* vs. [beigiŋ] *begging*, or in syllable-final position, e.g. [beik] *bake* vs. [beig] *beg*. These include differences in F_1 transition, duration of the closure interval, and duration of the preceding vowel (cf. Lisker, 1978).

Nasal consonants

The nasal consonants of English are [m n ŋ]. Similar to stop consonants, nasal consonants are produced with a closure in the supralaryngeal oral cavity. However, in contrast to stop consonants, the velum is open. Sound is propagated through the nose during the oral occlusion of a nasal consonant, and it is propagated through both the nose and mouth as the oral occlusion is released. There are several acoustic consequences of opening the nasal cavity in the production of a nasal consonant. A nasal "murmur" occurs prior to the release of the closure. This murmur has a spectrum dominated by a low frequency prominence usually around 250 Hz. In addition, the murmur has additional resonances above 700 Hz which have lower amplitudes. Another change in the spectrum is the presence of antiformants or *zeros*. Zeros selectively absorb acoustic energy, thus reducing the amplitude components at or near the antiresonant frequency (cf. Chapter 7 for further discussion).

The nasal murmur is not the same for nasal consonants varying in place of articulation (Fujimura, 1962). However, studies exploring the acoustic cues for nasal consonants have shown that the presence of a low frequency broadband murmur around 250 Hz preceding the onset of the formant transitions is sufficient for the perception of a nasal consonant irrespective of place of articulation (Cooper *et al.*, 1952).

The onset frequencies and direction of the formant transitions cue place of articulation in a manner similar to stop consonants. Thus, if a nasal murmur were synthesized preceding the onset of the formant transitions replacing the burst shown in Figure 10.2A, then the synthesized syllables will be perceived as [ma], [na] and the non-English syllable [ŋa] respectively. Although the fine details do differ, it is the case that the onset frequencies and direction of the formant transitions are similar for "homorganic" nasals and stops, i.e. nasals and stops that share the same place of articulation.

Liquids and glides

The sounds [l r] are called *liquids*, and the sounds [w y] are called *glides*. All of them are produced with a partial constriction in the vocal tract. Research on the acoustic cues for the perception of liquids and glides has shown that the rate, i.e. the duration, of the formant transitions provides the essential cue for these speech sounds (O'Connor *et al.*, 1957). In particular, if the formant transitions are about 40 milliseconds or longer, listeners will perceive a glide. If the transition durations are shorter, listeners may perceive stop consonants (Liberman *et al.*, 1956). Perception of glides and liquids are enhanced if the formant transitions remain at their onset formant frequencies for some 30 milliseconds or so before the transitions begin moving toward the steady-state formant frequencies of the vowel.

The perception of the particular liquid or glide, i.e. [l r w y], depends on the onset frequencies and direction of the formant transitions, particularly of the second and higher formants. For example, if the formant transitions are rising relative to the frequency of the vowel steady-state, the listener will perceive a [w]. In contrast, if F_2 is falling and F_3 is steady, listeners will perceive [l].

Fricatives

The acoustic cues for fricative consonants are quite complex and will only be briefly summarized. In English, the fricative consonants include [f θ s š v δ z ž]. Experiments using synthetic speech have shown that the primary acoustic cue to the fricative manner of articulation, irrespective of place of articulation and voicing, is the presence of aperiodic noise in the spectrum (Delattre, Liberman and Cooper 1962). The duration of this noise should be at least 20 milliseconds (Jongman, 1986). In natural speech, however, the duration of the fricative noise is considerably longer, of the order of 100 milliseconds. The onset of the noise must be fairly gradual. If it is too abrupt, the stimulus will be perceived as an affricate or a stop (Gerstman, 1957; Cutting and Rosner, 1974).

The overall amplitude of the noise and the distribution of spectral peaks contribute to the perception of the different places of articulation for fricative consonants. For example, both [s š] have overall greater amplitude than [f θ] (Strevens, 1960; Heinz and Stevens, 1961). Listeners' perception of fricative place of articulation is affected by varying the overall amplitude of the frication noise relative to that of the vowel. The same stimulus is perceived as [s] when the amplitude of the high frequency noise is greater than that of the vowel, but it is perceived as [θ] when the amplitude of the noise is lower than that of the vowel (Stevens, 1985). Moreover, if the major frequency peak of the noise is lowered from around 5 kHz to around 2.5 kHz, listeners' perception will change from [s] to [š] (Delattre *et al.*, 1964; Stevens, 1985).

Exercises

1. Review the acoustic cues for the perception of vowels. What are they? Compare the role of formant transitions and vowels.

2. How do the acoustic cues for stop consonants differ from those for nasal consonants? Do they share any attributes?

3. Is there one acoustic cue which corresponds to one phonetic segment? Discuss.

Bibliography

Abbs, J. H. (1986) Invariance and variability in speech production: A distinction between linguistic intent and its neuromotor implementation. *In* J. S. Perkell and D. H. Klatt (eds.), *Invariance and variability in speech processes*. Hillsdale, New Jersey, Erlbaum

Abramson, A. and Lisker, L. (1970) Discriminability along the voicing continuum: Cross-language tests. *Proceedings of the Sixth International Congress of Phonetic Sciences*. Prague: Academia

Armstrong, L. E. and Ward, I. C. (1926) *Handbook of English intonation*. Leipzig and Berlin: B. G. Teubner

Assmann, P. F. (1979) The role of context in vowel perception. Master's thesis, University of Alberta, Canada

Atal, B. S. and Hanauer, S. L. (1971) Speech analysis and synthesis by linear prediction of the speech wave, *Journal of the Acoustical Society of America* **50**, 637–55

Atkinson, J. R. (1973) Aspects of intonation in speech: Implications from an experimental study of fundamental frequency. Unpublished Ph.D. dissertation, University of Connecticut, Storrs

Baker, E., Blumstein, S. E. and Goodglass, H. (1981) Interaction between phonological and semantic factors in auditory comprehension, *Neuropsychologia* **19**, 1–16

Basso, A., Casati, G. and Vignolo, L. A. (1977) Phonemic identification defects in aphasia, *Cortex* **13**, 84–95

Bell, A. M. (1867) *Visible speech or self-interpreting physiological letters for the writing of all languages in one alphabet*. London: Simpkin and Marshall

Bell, C. G., Fujisaki, H., Heinz, J. M., Stevens, K. N. and House, A. S. (1961) Reduction of speech spectra by analysis-by-synthesis techniques, *Journal of the Acoustical Society of America* **33**, 1725–36

Bell-Berti, F. (1973) The velopharyngeal mechanism: An electromyographic study. Unpublished Ph.D. thesis, City University of New York; also Status Report on Speech Research, Supplement, Haskins Laboratories, 270 Crown Street, New Haven, Conn. 06510

Beranek, L. L. (1949) *Acoustics*. New York: McGraw-Hill

Bertoncini, J., Bijeljac-Babic, R., Blumstein, S. and Mehler, J. (1987) Discrimination in neonates of very short CVs, *Journal of the Acoustical Society of America* **82**, 31–7

Bladon, R. and Lindblom B. (1981) Modeling the judgement of vowel quality differences, *Journal of the Acoustical Society of America* **69**, 1414–22

Bloomfield, L. (1933) *Language*. New York: Holt

Blumstein, S. E. (1973) *A phonological investigation of aphasic speech*. The Hague: Mouton

Blumstein, S. E. and Stevens, K. N. (1979) Acoustic invariance in speech production: Evidence from measurements of the spectral characteristics of stop consonants, *Journal of the Acoustical Society of America* **66**, 1001–17

Blumstein, S. E. and Stevens, K. N. (1980) Perceptual invariance and onset spectra for stop consonants in different vowel environments, *Journal of the Acoustical Society of America* **67**, 648–62

Blumstein, S. E. and Stevens, K. N. (1981) Phonetic features and acoustic invariance in speech, *Cognition* **10**, 25–32

Blumstein, S. E., Baker, E. and Goodglass, E. (1977a) Phonological factors in auditory comprehension in aphasia, *Neuropsychologia* **15**, 19–36

Blumstein, S. E., Cooper, W. E., Zurif, E. and Caramazza, A. (1977b) The perception and production of voice-onset time in aphasia, *Neuropsychologia*, **15**, 371–83

Blumstein, S. E., Cooper, W. E., Goodglass, H., Statlender, S. and Gottlieb, J. (1980) Production deficits in aphasia: A voice-onset time analysis. *Brain and Language* **9**, 153–70

Blumstein, S. E., Tartter, V. C., Nigro, G. and Statlender, S. (1984) Acoustic cues for the perception of articulation in aphasia, *Brain and Language* **22**, 128–49

Bogert, C. M. (1960) The influence of sound on the behavior of amphibians and reptiles, *in* W. E. Lanyon and W. N. Tavoglga (eds.) *Animal sound and communication*, American Institute of Biological Sciences, Washington DC

Bolt, R. H., Cooper, F. S., David, E. E. Jr, Denes, P. B., Pickett, J. M. and Stevens, K. N. (1973) Speaker identification by speech spectrograms: Some further observations, *Journal of the Acoustical Society of America* **54**, 531–4

Bond, Z. S. (1976) Identification of vowels excerpted from neutral nasal contexts, *Journal of the Acoustical Society of America* **59**, 1229–32

Bosma, J. F. (1957) Deglutition: Pharyngeal stage, *Physiological Review* **37**, 275–300

Bouhuys, A. (1974) *Breathing*. New York: Grune and Stratton

Bouhuys, A., Proctor, D. F. and Mead, J. (1966) Kinetic aspect of singing, *Journal of Applied Physiology* **21**, 483–96

Bradshaw, J. L. and Nettleton, N. C. (1981) The nature of hemispheric specialization in man, *The Behavioral and Brain Sciences* **4**, 51–92

Broca, P. (1861) Nouvelle observation d'aphemie produite par une lesion de la motie posterieure des deuxieme et troisieme circonvolutions frontales, *Bulletin de la Societé d'Anatomique. Paris* **6** (series 2), 398–407

Bryden, P. (1982) *Laterality: Functional asymmetry in the intact brain*. New York: Academic Press

Capranica, R. R. (1965) *The evoked vocal response of the bullfrog*. Cambridge, Mass.: MIT Press

Chapin, C., Tseng, C. Y. and Lieberman, P. (1982) Short-term release cues for stop consonant place of articulation in child speech, *Journal of the Acoustical Society of America* **71**, 179–86

Chiba, T. and Kajiyama, J. (1941) *The vowel: Its nature and structure*. Tokyo: Tokyo-Kaiseikan Publishing Co.

Chomsky, N. (1957) *Syntactic structures*. The Hague: Mouton

Chomsky, N. and Halle, M. (1968) *The sound pattern of English*. New York: Harper and Row

Clark, H. H. and Clark, E. V. (1977) *Psychology and language*. New York: Harcourt Brace Jovanovich

Cole, R., Rudnicky, A. I., Zue, V. W. and Reddy, D. J. (1980) Speech as patterns on paper. *In* R. A. Cole (ed.), *Perception and production of fluent speech*. New York: Lawrence Erlbaum

Collier, R. (1975) Physiological correlates of intonation patterns, *Journal of the Acoustical Society of America* **58**, 249–55

Cooper, W. and Cooper, J. P. (1980) *Syntax and speech*. Cambridge, Mass.: Harvard University Press

Cooper, W. and Sorenson J. M. (1981) *Fundamental frequency in sentence production*. New York: Springer

Cooper, F. S., Delattre, P. C., Liberman, A. M., Borst, J. M. and Gerstman, L. J. (1952) Some experiments on the perception of synthetic speech sounds, *Journal of the Acoustical Society of America* **24**, 597–606

Crelin, E. S. (1969) *Anatomy of the newborn: An atlas*. Philadelphia: Lea and Febiger

Crelin, E. S. (1973) *Functional anatomy of the newborn*. New Haven: Yale University Press

229

Cutting, J. E. (1972) Plucks and bows are categorically perceived, sometimes, *Perception and Psychophysics* **31**, 462–76

Cutting, J. E. (1974) Two left hemisphere mechanisms in speech perception, *Perception and Psychophysics* **16**, 601–12

Cutting, J. E. and Eimas, P. D. (1975) Phonetic analysers and processing of speech in infants. *In* J. F. Kavanagh and J. E. Cutting (eds.), *The role of speech in language*. Cambridge, Mass.: MIT Press

Cutting, J. and Rosner, B. (1974) Categories and boundaries in speech and music, *Perception and Psychophysics* **16**, 564–70

Daniloff, R. and Moll, K. (1968) Coarticulation of lip rounding, *Journal of Speech and Hearing Research* **11**, 707–21

Darwin, C. (1859) *On the origin of species*. Facsimile ed. 1964. Cambridge, Mass.: Harvard University Press

Deacon, T. W. (1985) Connections of the inferior periarcuate area in the brain of *Macaca fascicularis*: An experimental and comparative neuroanatomical investigation of language circuitry and its evolution. Ph.D. dissertation, Harvard University

Dejours, P. (1963) Control of respiration by arterial chemoreceptors, *in Regulation of Respiration, Annals of The New York Academy of Sciences* **109**, 682–95

Delattre, P. C. (1968) Divergences entre la nasalité vocalique et consonantique en français, *Word* **24**, 64–72

Delattre, P. C., Liberman, A. M., and Cooper, F. S. (1955) Acoustic loci and transitional cues for consonants, *Journal of the Acoustical Society of America* **27**, 769–73

Delattre, P. C., Liberman, A. M., and Cooper, F. S. (1962) Formant transitions and loci as acoustic correlates of place of articulation in American fricatives, *Studia Linguistica* **16**, 104–21

Delattre, P., Liberman, A. M., Cooper, F. S. and Gerstman, L. J. (1952) An experimental study of the acoustic determinants of vowel color: Observations on one- and two-formant vowels synthesized from spectrographic patterns, *Word* **8**, 195–210

Delgutte, B. (1980) Representation of speech-like sounds in the discharge patterns of auditory-nerve fibers, *Journal of the Acoustical Society of America* **68**, 843–57

Denes, P. (1955) Effect of duration on the perception of voicing, *Journal of the Acoustical Society of America* **27**, 761–4

Dorman, M., Studdert–Kennedy, M. and Raphael, L. (1977) The invariance problem in initial voiced stops: Release bursts and formant transitions as functionally equivalent context-dependent cues, *Perception and Psychophysics* **22**, 109–22

Draper, M. H., Ladefoged, P. and Whitteridge, D. (1960) Expiratory pressures and air flow during speech, *British Medical Journal* **1**, 1837–43

Dudley, H. (1936) Synthesizing speech, *Bell Laboratories Record* **15**, 98–102

Dudley, H. (1939) The Vocoder, *Bell Laboratories Record* **17**, 122–6

Dudley, H., Reisz, R. R. and Watkins, S. S. A. (1939) A synthetic speaker, *Journal of the Franklin Institute* **227**, 739–64

Dunn, H. K. 1950. The calculation of vowel resonances and an electrical vocal tract, *Journal of the Acoustical Society of America,* **22**, 740–53

Eimas, P. D., Siqueland, E. R., Jusczyk, P. and Vigorito, J. (1971) Speech perception in infants, *Science* **171**, 303–6

Erikson, D. (1975) A laryngeal description of Thai tones, unpublished paper presented at Annual Meeting of the Linguistic Society of America, San Francisco.

Evarts, E. V. (1973) Motor cortex reflexes associated with learned movement, *Science* **179**, 501–3

Fairbanks, G. and Grubb, P. (1961) A psychological investigation of vowel formants, *Journal of Speech and Hearing Research* **4**, 203–19

Fant, G. (1956) On the predictability of formant levels and spectrum envelopes from formant frequencies. *In* M. Halle, H. Lunt and H. MacLean (eds.), *For Roman Jakobson*. The Hague: Mouton

Fant, G. (1960) *Acoustic theory of speech production*. The Hague: Mouton

Fant, G. (1966) A note on vocal tract size patterns and non-uniform *F*-pattern scalings, *Quarterly Progress Status Report*. Stockholm: Speech Transmission Laboratory, Royal Institute of Technology

Fant, G. (1969) Distinctive features and phonetic dimensions, STL-QPSR 2-3/1969; also pp. 1–18 in Fant, G. (1973) *Speech, sounds and features*. Cambridge, Mass.: MIT Press

Fant, G. (1973) *Speech, sounds and features*. Cambridge, Mass.: MIT Press

Ferrein, C. J. (1741) *Mémoires de l'Académie des Sciences des Paris*, November 15, 409–32

Fischer-Jorgensen, E. (1972) Perceptual studies of Danish stop consonants, *Annual Report of Institute of Phonetics, University of Copenhagen* **6**, 75–168

Flanagan, J. L. (1955a) A difference limen for vowel formant frequency, *Journal of the Acoustical Society of America* **27**, 306–10

Flanagan, J. L. (1955b) Difference limen for the intensity of a vowel sound, *Journal of the Acoustical Society of America* **27**, 613–17

Flanagan, J. L. (1957) Note on the design of "terminal analog" speech synthesizers, *Journal of the Acoustical Society of America* **29**, 306–10

Flanagan, J. L. (1972) *Speech analysis, synthesis and perception*. 2nd ed. Springer, New York, Heidelberg, Berlin

Flanagan, J. L., Ishizaka, K. and Shipley, K. L. (1975) Synthesis of speech from a dynamic model of the vocal cords and vocal tract, *Bell System Technical Journal* **54**, 485–506

Flanagan, J. L., Coker, C. H., Rabiner, L. R., Schafer, R. W. and Umeda, N. (1970) Synthetic voices for computers, *IEEE spectrum* **7**, 22–45

Flege, J. E. (1984) The detection of French accent by American listeners, *Journal of the Acoustical Society of America* **76**, 692–707

Fletcher, H. (1940) Auditory patterns, *Journal of the Acoustical Society of America* **12**, 47–65

Folkins, J. W. (1985) Issues in speech motor control and their relation to the speech of individuals with cleft palate, *Cleft Palate Journal* **22**, 106–22

Folkins, J. W. and Zimmerman, G. N. (1981) Jaw-muscle activity during speech with the mandible fixed, *Journal of the Acoustical Society of America* **69**, 1441–4

Fowler, C. and Shankweiler, D. P. (1978) Identification of vowels in speech and non-speech contexts, *Journal of the Acoustical Society of America* **63**, suppl. I, S4 (A)

Fowler, C. and Smith, M. R. (1985) Speech perception as "vector analysis": An approach to the problems of invariance and segmentation. *In* J. Perkell, G. Fant, B. Lindblom, D. Klatt and S. Shattuck-Hufnagel (eds.), *Invariance and variability of speech processes*. New Jersey: Erlbaum

Freeman, F. J., Sands, E. S. and Harris, K. S. (1978) Temporal coordination of phonation and articulation in a case of verbal apraxia: A voice-onset time study, *Brain and Language* **6**, 106–11

Frishkopf, L. S. and Goldstein, M. H. Jr (1963) Responses to acoustic stimuli from single units in the eighth nerve of the bullfrog, *Journal of the Acoustical Society of America* **35**, 1219–28

Fromkin, V. A. (1971) The non-anomalous nature of anomalous utterances, *Language* **47**, 27–52

Fromkin, V. A. (ed.) (1973) *Speech errors as linguistic evidence*. The Hague: Mouton

Fry, D. B. (1955) Duration and intensity as physical correlates of linguistic stress, *Journal of the Acoustical Society of America* **35**, 765–9

Fujimura, O. (1962) Analysis of nasal consonants, *Journal of the Acoustical Society of America* **34**, 1865–75

Fujimura, I., Tatsumi, I. F. and Kagaya, R. (1973) Computational processing of palatographic patterns, *Journal of Phonetics* **1**, 47–54

Gandour, J. and Dardarananda, R. (1984) Voice onset time in aphasia: Thai II. Production, *Brain and Language* **23**, 177–205

Bibliography

Garding, E., Fujimura, O. and Hirose, H. (1970) Laryngeal control of Swedish word tones, a preliminary report of an EMG study, *Annual Bulletin of The Research Institute of Logopedics and Phonetics, University of Tokyo* **4**, 45–54

Gay, T. (1974) A cinefluorographic study of vowel production, *Journal of Phonetics* **2**, 255–66

Gerstman, L. (1957) Cues for distinguishing among fricatives, affricates and stop consonants. Unpublished doctoral dissertation, New York University.

Geschwind, N. (1965) Disconnection syndromes in animals and man, Part I, *Brain* **88**, 237–94; Part II, *Brain* **88**, 585–644

Gold, B. (1962) Computer program for pitch extraction, *Journal of the Acoustical Society of America* **34**, 916–21

Goldhor R. S. (1984) The effect of auditory transformations on speech. Sc.D. dissertation, Massachusetts Institute of Technology

Goldstein, U. G. (1980) An articulatory model for the vocal tracts of growing children. Sc.D. dissertation, Massachusetts Institute of Technology

Gracco, V. and Abbs, J. (1985) Dynamic control of the perioral system during speech: Kinematic analysis of autogenic and nonautogenic sensorimotor processes, *Journal of Neurophysiology* **54**, 418–32

Greenberg, J. (1963) *Universals of language*. Cambridge, Mass.: MIT Press

Greenberg, J. (1966) *Language universals*. The Hague: Mouton

Greenewalt, C. H. (1968) *Bird song: Acoustics and physiology*. Washington DC: Smithsonian Institute

Greenwood, D. D. (1961) Critical bandwidths and frequency co-ordinates of the basilar membrane, *Journal of the Acoustical Society of America* **33**, 1344–56

Hadding-Koch, K. (1961) *Acoustico-phonetic studies in the intonation of southern Swedish*. Lund, Sweden: C. W. K. Gleerup

Haggard, M. P., Ambler, S. and Callow, M. (1970) Pitch as a voicing cue, *Journal of the Acoustical Society of America* **47**, 613–17

Halle, M. and Stevens, K. N. (1959) Analysis by synthesis. *In* W. Wathen-Dunn and L. E. Woods (eds.), *Proceedings of the seminar on speech compression and processing*, AFCRC-TR-59-198, December 1959, vol. II, paper D7

Harris, K. S. (1974) Physiological aspects of articulatory behavior. *In* T. Sebeok (ed.), *Current trends in linguistics, vol. 12*. The Hague: Mouton

Hawkins, S. and Stevens, K. N. (1985) Acoustic and perceptual correlates of the non-nasal–nasal distinction for vowels, *Journal of the Acoustical Society of America* **77**, 1560–75

Hecker, M. H. L. and Kreul, E. J. (1971) Descriptions of the speech of patients with cancer of the vocal folds, Part 1: Measurements of fundamental frequency, *Journal of the Acoustical Society of America* **49**, 1275–82

Heinz, J. M. (1962) Reduction of speech spectra to descriptions in terms of vocal tract area functions. Unpublished Sc.D. thesis, Massachusetts Institute of Technology

Heinz, J. M. and Stevens, K. N. (1961) On the properties of voiceless fricative consonants, *Journal of the Acoustical Society of America* **33**, 589–96

Hellwag, C. (1781) *De Formatione Loquelae*. Dissertation, Tubingen

Henke, W. L. (1966) Dynamic articulatory model of speech production using computer simulation. Unpublished Sc.D. dissertation, Massachusetts Institute of Technology

Hermann, L. (1894) Nachtrag zur Untersuchung der Vocalcurven, *Arch. ges. Physiol.* **58**, 264–79

Hillenbrand, J. (1984) Speech perception by infants: Categorization based on nasal place of articulation. *Journal of the Acoustical Society of America* **75**, 1613–22

Hirose, H. and Ushijama, T. (1974) The function of the posterior cricoarytenoid in speech articulation, *Status Report on Speech Research* SR 37/38, January–June 1974, 94–102, Haskins Laboratories, 370 Crown St, New Haven, Conn.

232

Hirsch, I. J. (1959) Auditory perception of temporal order, *Journal of the Acoustical Society of America* **31**, 759–67

Hirsch, I. J. and Sherrick, C. E. Jr (1961) Perceived order in different sense modalities, *Journal of Experimental Psychology* **62**, 423–32

Hixon, T., Goldman, M. and Mead, J. (1973) Kinematics of the chest wall during speech production: Volume displacements of the rib cage, abdomen, and lung, *Journal of Speech and Hearing Research* **16**, 78–115

Hollien, H. (1962) Vocal fold thickness and fundamental frequency of phonation, *Journal of Speech and Hearing Research* **5**, 237–43

Hollien, H. and Colton, R. H. (1969) Four laminographic studies of vocal fold thickness, *Folia Phoniatrica* **21**, 179–98

Hollien, H. and Curtis, J. F. (1960) A laminographic study of vocal pitch, *Speech and Hearing Research* **3**, 361–70

Holmes, J. N., Mattingly, I. G. and Shearme, J. N. (1964) Speech synthesis by rule, *Language and Speech* **1**, 127–43

Houde, R. (1967) *A study of tongue body movement during selected speech*, Speech Communications Research Laboratory Monograph No. 2, Santa Barbara, Calif.

House, A. S. and Stevens, K. N. (1956) Analog studies of the nasalization of vowels, *Journal of Speech and Hearing Disorders* **21**, 218–32

Hoy, R. R. and Paul, R. C. (1973) Genetic control of song specificity in crickets, *Science* **180**, 82–3

Itoh, M., Sasanuma, S. and Ushijima, T. (1979) Velar movements during speech in a patient with apraxia of speech, *Brain and Language* **7**, 227–39

Itoh, M., Sasanuma, S., Tatsumi, I. F., Murakami, S., Fukusako, Y. and Suzuki, T. (1982) Voice onset time characteristics in apraxia of speech, *Brain and Language* **17**, 193–210

Jakobson, R (1968) (transl. A. R. Keiler) *Child language, aphasia and phonological universals.* The Hague: Mouton

Jakobson, R. and Waugh, L. R. (1979) *The sound shape of language.* Bloomington: Indiana University Press

Jakobson R., Fant, G. M. and Halle, M. (1963) *Preliminaries to speech analysis.* Cambridge, Mass.: MIT Press

Jauhianen, T. and Nuutila, Λ. (1977) Auditory perception of speech and speech sounds in recent and recovered cases of aphasia, *Brain and Language* **6**, 47–51

Jones, D. (1919) X-ray photographs of the cardinal vowels, *Proceedings of the Royal Institute* **22**, 12–13

Jones, D. (1932) *An outline of English phonetics.* New York: E. P. Dutton.

Jongman, A. (1986) Duration of frication noise as a perceptual cue to place and manner of articulation in English fricatives. Under editorial review.

Joos, M. (1948) Acoustic phonetics, *Language* **24**, Suppl., 1–136

Jusczyk, (1986) A review of speech perception research. *In* L. Kaufman, J. Thomas and K. Boff (eds.), *Handbook of perception and performance.* New York: Wiley

Kahn, D. (1978) On the identification of isolated vowels, *UCLA Working Papers in Phonetics* **41**, 26–31

Katz, W. (1986) An acoustic and perceptual investigation of co-articulation in aphasia. Unpublished doctoral dissertation, Brown University

Katz, W. and Blumstein, S. E. (1987) Acoustic properties for the perception of nasal manner of articulation. Manuscript.

Keating, P. J. and Blumstein, S. E. (1978) Effects of transition length on the perception of stop consonants, *Journal of the Acoustical Society of America* **64**, 57–64

Keating, P. J. and Buhr, R. (1978) Fundamental frequency in the speech of infants and children, *Journal of the Acoustical Society of America* **63**, 567–71

Kent, R. D. and Rosenbek, J. C. (1983) Acoustic patterns of apraxia of speech, *Journal of Speech and Hearing Research* **26**, 231–49

Kersta, K. G. (1962) Voiceprint identification, *Nature* **196**, 1253–7

Kewley-Port, D. (1983) Time-varying features as correlates of place of articulation in stop consonants, *Journal of the Acoustical Society of America* **73**, 322–35

Kewley-Port, D., Pisoni, D. B. and Studdert-Kennedy, M. (1983) Perception of static and dynamic acoustic cues to place of articulation in initial stop consonants, *Journal of the Acoustical Society of America* **73**, 1779–93

Kimura, D. (1961) Some effects of temporal lobe damage on auditory perception, *Canadian Journal of Psychology* **15**, 156–65

Kimura, D. (1967) Functional asymmetry of the brain in dichotic listening, *Cortex* **3**, 163–78

Kirchner, J. A. (1970) *Pressman and Kelemen's physiology of the larynx*, rev. ed. Washington DC: American Academy of Opthamology and Otolaryngology

Klatt, D. H. (1973) Interaction between two factors that influence vowel duration, *Journal of the Acoustical Society of America* **54**, 1102–4

Klatt, D.H. (1976) Linguistic uses of segmental duration in English: Acoustical and perceptual evidence, *Journal of the Acoustical Society of America* **59**, 1208–21

Klatt, D. H. (1980) Software for a cascade/parallel formant synthesizer, *Journal of the Acoustical Society of America* **67**, 971–95

Klatt, D. H., Stevens, K. N. and Mead, J. (1968) Studies of articulatory activity and airflow during speech, *Annals of the New York Academy of Sciences* **155**, 42–54

Koenig, W., Dunn, H. K. and Lacey, L. Y. (1946) The sound spectrograph, *Journal of the Acoustical Society of America* **18**, 19–49

Kratzenstein, C. G. (1780) Sur la naissance de la formation des voyelles, *Journal of Physiology* **21** (1782), 358–81 (translated from *Acta Academic Petrograd*)

Kuehn, D. P. and Tomblin, J. B. (1977) A cineradiographic investigation of children's w/r substitutions, *Journal of Speech and Hearing Disorders* **42**, 462–73

Kuhl, P. K. (1979a) The perception of speech in early infancy. *In* N. J. Lass (ed.), *Speech and language: Advances in basic research and practice (Vol. 1)*. New York: Academic Press

Kuhl, P. K. (1979b) Speech perception in early infancy: Perceptual constancy for spectrally dissimilar vowel categories, *Journal of the Acoustical Society of America* **66**, 1668–79

Kuhl, P. K. (1980) Perceptual constancy for speech-sound categories in early infancy. *In* G. H. Yeni-Komshian, J. F. Kavanagh and C. A. Ferguson (eds.), *Child phonology: Perception (Vol. 2)*. New York: Academic Press

Kuhl, P. K. (1981) Discrimination of speech by nonhuman animals: Basic auditory sensitivities conducive to the perception of speech-sound categories, *Journal of the Acoustical Society of America* **70**, 340–9

Kuhl, P. K., 1983. Perception of auditory equivalence classes for speech in early infancy. *Infant Behavior and Development*, **6**, 263–85

Kuhl, P. K. and Miller, J. D. (1974) Discrimination of speech sounds by the chinchilla: /t/ vs /d/ in CV syllables, *Journal of the Acoustical Society of America* **56**, Suppl. 2, S217

Kuhl, P. K. and Miller, J. D. (1975) Speech perception by the chinchilla: Voiced–voiceless distinction in alveolar plosive consonants, *Science* **190**, 69–72

Kuhl, P. K. and Miller, J. D. (1982) Discrimination of auditory target dimensions in the presence or absence of variation in a second dimension by infants, *Perception and Psychophysics* **32**, 279–92

Kurowski, K. and Blumstein, S. E. (1984) Perceptual integration of the murmur and formant transitions for place of articulation in nasal consonants, *Journal of the Acoustical Society of America* **76**, 383–90

Ladefoged, P. (1971) *Preliminaries to linguistic phonetics*. Chicago: Chicago University Press

Ladefoged, P. (1975) *A course in phonetics*. New York: Harcourt Brace Jovanovich

Ladefoged, P. and Broadbent, D. E. (1957) Information conveyed by vowels, *Journal of the Acoustical Society of America* **29**, 98–104

Ladefoged, P., DeClerk, J., Lindau, M. and Papcun, G. (1972) An auditory motor theory of speech production, *UCLA Phonetics Laboratory, Working Papers in Phonetics* **22**, 48–76

Laitman, J. T. and Heimbuch, R. C. (1982) The basicranium of Plio-Pleistocene hominids as an indicator of their upper respiratory systems, *American Journal of Physical Anthropology* **51**, 15–34

Laitman, J. T., Crelin, E. S. and Conlogue, G. J. (1977) The function of the epiglottis in monkey and man, *Yale Journal of Biology and Medicine* **50**, 43–8

La Mettrie, J. O. (1747) *De l'homme machine*. A. Vartainina (ed.), critical ed. 1960. Princeton: Princeton University Press

Landahl, K. (1982) The onset of structural discourse; a developmental study of the acquisition of language. Ph.D. dissertation, Brown University

Landahl, K. and Gould, H. J. (1986) Congenital malformation of the speech tract: Preliminary investigation and model development. Proceedings of the Association for Research in Otolaryngology, 1986 meeting.

Lane, H. (1965) The motor theory of speech perception: A critical review, *Psychological Review* **72**, 275–309

Lawrence, W. 1953. The synthesis of speech from signals that have a low information rate. *In* W. Jackson (ed.), *Communication theory*, London: Butterworths Sci. Pub.

LeFrancois, R., Gautier, H., Pasquis, P. and Bargas, E. (1969) Factors controlling respiration during muscular exercise at altitude, *Proceedings of the Federation of American Societies for Experimental Biology* **28**, 1298–1300

Lehiste, I. (1961) Some acoustic correlates of accent in Serbo-Croatian, *Phonetica* **7**, 114–47

Lenneberg, E. H. (1967) *Biological foundations of language*. New York: Wiley

Lettvin, J. Y., Maturana, H. R., McCulloch, W. S. and Pitts, W. H. (1959) What the frog's eye tells the frog's brain, *Proceedings of the Institute of Radio Engineers* **47**, 1940–51

Liberman, A. M. (1970a) The grammars of speech and language, *Cognitive Psychology* **1**, 301–23

Liberman, A. M. (1970b) Some characteristics of perception in the speech mode, *Perception and Its Disorders* **48**, 238–54

Liberman, A. M. and Mattingly, I. G. (1985) The motor theory of speech revised, *Cognition* **21**, 1–36

Liberman, A. M., Cooper, F. S. Shankweiler, D. P. and Studdert-Kennedy, M. (1967) Perception of the speech code, *Psychological Review* **74**, 431–61

Liberman, A. M., Delattre, P. C., Gerstman, L. J. and Cooper, F. S. (1956) Tempo of frequency change as a cue for distinguishing classes of speech sounds, *Journal of Experimental Psychology* **52**, 127–37

Lieberman, P. (1960) Some acoustic correlates of word stress in American English, *Journal of the Acoustical Society of America* **33**, 451–4

Lieberman, P. (1961) Perturbations in vocal pitch, *Journal of the Acoustical Society of America* **33**, 597–603

Lieberman, P. (1963) Some acoustic measures of the fundamental periodicity of normal and pathological larynges, *Journal of the Acoustical Society of America* **35**, 344–53

Lieberman, P. (1965) On the acoustic basis of the perception of intonation by linguists, *Word* **21**, 40–54

Lieberman, P. (1967) *Intonation, perception, and language*. Cambridge, Mass.: MIT Press

Lieberman, P. (1968) Direct comparison of subglottal and esophageal pressure during speech, *Journal of the Acoustical Society of America* **43**, 1157–64

Lieberman, P. (1970) Towards a unified phonetic theory, *Linguistic Inquiry* **1**, 307–22

Lieberman, P. (1973) On the evolution of language: A unified view, *Cognition* **2**, 59–94

Bibliography

Lieberman, P. (1975) *On the origins of language: An introduction to the evolution of human speech*. New York: Macmillan.

Lieberman, P. (1976) Phonetic features and physiology: A reappraisal, *Journal of Phonetics* **4**, 91–112

Lieberman, P. (1980) On the development of vowel production in young children. *In* G. Yeni-Komshian and J. Kavanaugh (eds.), *Child phonology: Perception and production*, pp. 113–142. New York: Academic Press

Lieberman, P. (1984) *The biology and evolution of language*. Cambridge, Mass.: Harvard University Press

Lieberman, P. and Crelin, E. S. (1971) On the speech of Neanderthal man, *Linguistic Inquiry* **2**, 203–22

Lieberman, M. R. and Lieberman, P. (1973) Olson's "projective verse" and the use of breath control as a structural element, *Language and Style* **5**, 287–98

Lieberman, P. and Michaels, S. B. (1963) On the discrimination of missing pitch pulses, *Proceedings of the Speech Communications Seminar*. Stockholm: Royal Institute of Technology

Lieberman, P., Crelin, E. S. and Klatt, D. H. (1972) Phonetic ability and related anatomy of the newborn, adult human, Neanderthal man, and the chimpanzee, *American Anthropologist* **74**, 287–307

Lieberman, P., Knudson, R. and Mead, J. (1969) Determination of the rate of change of fundamental frequency with respect to subglottal air pressure during sustained phonation, *Journal of the Acoustical Society of America* **45**, 1537–43

Lieberman, P., Landahl, K. and Ryalls, J. H. (1982) Sentence intonation in British and American English, *Journal of the Acoustical Society of America* **71**, Suppl. I, S112

Lieberman, P., Katz, W., Jongman, A., Zimmerman, R. and Miller, M. (1985) Measures of the sentence intonation of read and spontaneous speech in American English, *Journal of the Acoustical Society of America* **77**, 649–57

Lifschitz, S. (1933) Two integral laws of sound perception relating loudness and apparent duration of sound impulses, *Journal of the Acoustical Society of America* **7**, 213–19

Liljencrants, J. and Lindblom, B. (1972) Numerical simulation of vowel quality systems: The role of perceptual contrast, *Language* **48**, 839–62

Lindau, M., Jacobson, L. and Ladefoged, P. (1972) The feature advanced tongue root, *UCLA Phonetics Laboratory, Working Papers in Phonetics* **22**, 76–94

Lindblom, B. (1971) Phonetics and the description of language. *In* A. Rigault and R. Charbonneau (eds.), *Proceedings of the VIIth International Congress of Phonetic Sciences, Montreal*

Lindblom, B., Lubker, J. and Gay, T. (1979) Formant frequencies of some fixed-mandible vowels and a model of speech motor programming by predictive simulation, *Journal of Phonetics* **7**, 147–61

Lisker, L. (1978) *Rapid* vs. *Rabid*: A catalogue of acoustic features that may cue the distinction. *Status Report on Speech Research* **SR-54**, 127–32

Lisker, L. and Abramson, A. S. (1964) A cross-language study of voicing in initial stops: acoustical measurements, *Word* **20**, 384–422

Lisker, L. and Abramson, A. S. (1971) Distinctive features and laryngeal control, *Language* **47**, 767–85

Lisker, L., Cooper, F. S. and Schvey, M. H. (1969) Transillumination of the larynx in running speech, *Journal of the Acoustical Society of America* **45**, 1544–6

Lisker, L., Liberman, A. M., Erickson, D. M., Dechovitz, D. and Mandler, R. (1977) On pushing the voice onset time (VOT) boundary about, *Language and Speech* **20**, 209–16

Lubker, J. and Gay, T. (1982) Anticipatory labial coarticulation: Experimental, biological and linguistic variables, *Journal of the Acoustical Society of America* **71**, 437–48

236

Lubker, J. F., Fritzell, B. and Lindquist, J. (1970) Velopharyngeal function: An electro-myographic study, *Speech Transmission Laboratory*, Royal Institute of Technology, Stockholm, QPSR 4, 9–20

Luria, A. R. (1961) The pathology of directive function of speech, *Reports at the VIIth International Congress of Neurology, Rome*, pp. 601–3. The Hague: Mouton

Mack, M. A. (1983) Psycholinguistic consequences of early bilingualism: A comparative study of the performance of English monolinguals and French–English bilinguals in phonetics, syntax, and semantics experiments. Unpublished Ph.D. dissertation, Brown University

Mack, M. and Blumstein, S. E. (1983) Further evidence of acoustic invariance in speech production: The stop-glide contrast, *Journal of the Acoustical Society of America* **73**, 1739–50

Mack, M. and Lieberman, P. (1985) Acoustic analysis of words produced by a child from 46 to 149 weeks, *Journal of Child Language* **12**, 527–50

MacLean, P. D. (1985) Evolutionary psychiatry and the triune brain, *Psychological Medicine* **15**, 219–21

MacNeilage, P. F. (1970) Motor control of serial ordering in speech, *Psychological Review* **77**, 182–96

MacNeilage, P. F. and DeClerk, J. L. (1969) On the motor control of coarticulation in CVC monosyllables, *Journal of the Acoustical Society of America* **45**, 1217–33

Maeda, S. (1976) A characterization of American English intonation. Sc.D. thesis, Massachusetts Institute of Technology.

Mattingly, I. G., Liberman, A. M., Syrdal, A. K. and Halwes, T. (1971) Discrimination in speech and nonspeech modes, *Cognitive Psychology* **2**, 131–57

Mayr, E. (1982) *The growth of biological thought: Diversity, evolution, and inheritance*. Cambridge, Mass.: Harvard University Press

McAdam, D. W. and Whitaker, H. A. (1971) Language production: Electroencephalographic localization in the normal human brain, *Science* **172**, 499–502

Mead, J., Bouhays, A. and Proctor, D. F. (1968) Mechanisms generating subglottic pressure, *Sound Production in Man, Annals of the New York Academy of Sciences* **155**, 177–81

Miceli, G., Caltagirone, C., Gainotti, C. and Payer-Rigo, P. (1978) Discrimination of voice versus place contrasts in aphasia, *Brain and Language* **6**, 47–51

Miceli, G., Gainotti, G., Caltagirone, C. and Masullo, C. (1980) Some aspects of phonological impairment in aphasia, *Brain and Language* **11**, 159–69

Miles, F. A. and Evarts, E. V. (1979) Concepts of motor organization, *Annual Review of Physiology* **30**, 327–62

Miller, G. A. (1956) The magical number seven, plus or minus two: Some limits in our capacity for processing information, *Psychological Review* **63**, 81–97

Miller, G. A. and Nicely, P. E. (1955) An analysis of perceptual confusions among some English consonants, *Journal of the Acoustical Society of America* **27**, 338–52

Miller, J. D. (1981) Effects of speaking rate on segmental distinctions. In P. D. Eimas and J. L. Miller (eds.), *Perspectives in the study of speech*. New Jersey: Erlbaum Press.

Minifie, F. D., Hixon, T. J., Kelsey, A. A. and Woodhouse, R. J. (1970) Lateral pharyngeal wall movement during speech production, *Journal of Speech and Hearing Research* **13**, 584–94

Minifie, F. D., Kelsey, C. A. and Hixon, T. J. (1968) Measurement of vocal fold motion using an ultrasonic Doppler velocity monitor, *Journal of the Acoustical Society of America* **43**, 1165–9

Molfese, D. L. (1972) Cerebral asymmetry in infants, children, and adults: Auditory evoked responses to speech and noise stimuli. Unpublished Ph.D. dissertation, Pennsylvania State University

Morse, P. A. (1972) The discrimination of speech and nonspeech stimuli in early infancy, *Journal of Experimental Child Psychology* **14**, 477–92

Morton, J. and Jassem, W. (1965) Acoustic correlates of stress, *Language and Speech* **8**, 159–81

Bibliography

Müller, J. (1848) *The physiology of the senses, voice, and muscular motion with the mental faculties* (W. Baly, trans.). London: Walton and Maberly

Nearey, T. (1976) Features for vowels. Unpublished Ph.D. dissertation, University of Connecticut, Storrs

Nearey, T. (1978) *Phonetic features for vowels*. Bloomington, Indiana: Indiana University Linguistics Club

Negus, V. E. (1949) *The comparative anatomy and physiology of the larynx*. New York: Hafner

O'Connor, J. D., Gerstman, L. J., Liberman, A. M., Delattre, P. C. and Cooper, F. S. (1957) Acoustic cues for the perception of initial /w,y,r,l/ in English, *Word* **13**, 24–43

Ohala, J. (1966) A new photoelectric glottograph, *UCLA Phonetics Laboratory, Working Papers in Phonetics* **4**, 40–52

Ohala, J. (1970) Aspects of the control and production of speech, *UCLA Phonetics Laboratory, Working Papers in Phonetics* **15**

Ohala, J., and Hirose, H. (1970) The function of the sternohyoid muscle in speech, *Annual Bulletin of the Research Institute of Logopedics and Phoniatrics, University of Tokyo* **4**, 41–4

Ohman, S. E. G. (1966) Coarticulation in VCV utterances: Spectrographic measurements, *Journal of the Acoustical Society of America* **39**, 151–68

Penfield, W. and Roberts, L. (1959) *Speech and brain-mechanisms underlying language*. Princeton, NJ: Princeton University Press

Perkell, J. S. (1969) *Physiology of speech production: Results and implications of a quantitative cineradiographic study*. Cambridge, Mass.: MIT Press

Peterson, G. E. (1951) The phonetic value of vowels, *Language* **27**, 541–53

Peterson, G. E. and Barney, H. L. (1952) Control methods used in a study of the vowels, *Journal of the Acoustical Society of America* **24**, 175–84

Peterson, G. E. and Lehiste, I. (1960) Duration of syllable nuclei in English, *Journal of the Acoustical Society of America* **32**, 693–703

Peterson, G. E., Wang, W. S-Y., and Sivertson, E. (1958) Segmentation techniques in speech synthesis, *Journal of the Acoustical Society of America* **30**, 739–42

Piaget, J. (1980) *In* M. Piattelli-Palmarini (ed.), *Language and learning; the debate between Jean Piaget and Noam Chomsky*, pp. 107–30. Cambridge, Mass.: Harvard University Press

Pierrehumbert, J. (1979) The perception of fundamental frequency declination, *Journal of the Acoustical Society of America* **66**, 363–9

Pinker, S. (1984) *Language learnability and language development*. Cambridge, Mass.: Harvard University Press

Pisoni, D. B., Carrell, T. D. and Simnick, S. S. (1979) Does a listener need to recover the dynamic vocal tract gestures of a talker to recognise his vowels? *In* J. J. Wolf and D. H. Klatt (eds.). *Speech Communication Papers 1*. New York: Acoustical Society of America

Polit, A. and Bizzi, E. (1978) Processes controlling arm movements in monkeys, *Science* **201**, 1235–7

Pollack, I. (1952) The information of elementary audio displays, *Journal of the Acoustical Society of America* **24**, 745–9

Port, D. K. and Preston, M. S. (1972) Early apical stop production: A voice onset time study, *Haskins Laboratories Status Report on Speech Research* **29/30**, 125–49

Potter, R. K. and Steinberg, J. C. (1950) Toward the specification of speech, *Journal of the Acoustical Society of America* **22**, 807–20

Potter, R. K., Kopp, G. A. and Green, H. C. (1947) *Visible speech*. New York: D. Van Nostrand

Proctor, D. F. (1964) Physiology of the upper airway. *In* W. O. Fenn and H. Rahn (eds.), *Handbook of physiology, respiration, vol. 1*. Washington, DC: American Physiological Society

Purkinje, K (1836) *Badania w przedmiocie fizylolgil mowvy Ludzkiej*, Krakow

Rabiner, L. R. and Schafer, J. (1979) *Digital processing of speech*. New York: McGraw-Hill

Remez, R. E., Rubin, P. E. and Nygaard, L. C. (1986) On spontaneous speech and fluently spoken text: Production differences and perceptual distinctions, *Journal of the Acoustical Society of America* **78**, Suppl. 1, (A)

Remez, R. E., Rubin, P. E., Pisoni, D. P. and Carrell, T. O. (1981) Speech perception without traditional speech cues, *Science* **212**, 947–50

Repp, B. H. (1979) Relative amplitude of aspiration noise as a cue for syllable-initial stop consonants, *Language and Speech* **22**, 173–9

Repp, B. H. (1986) Perception of the [m]-[n] distinction in CV syllables, *Journal of the Acoustical Society of America* **79**, 1987–99

Robb, M. P. and Saxman, J. H. (1985) Developmental trends in vocal fundamental frequency of young children, *Journal of Speech and Hearing Research* **28**, 421–7

Rosen, G. (1958) Dynamic analog speech synthesizer, *Journal of the Acoustical Society of America* **30**, 201–9

Rothenberg, M. (1981) An interactive model for the voice source. STL-QPSR 4, 1–17, Stockholm Sweden, Speech Transmission Laboratory, Royal Institute of Technology

Rousselot, P. J. (1901) *Principes de phonetique experimentale*. Paris: H. Welter

Russell, G. O. (1928) *The vowel*. Columbus, Ohio: Ohio State University Press

Ryalls, J. (1986) An acoustic study of vowel production in aphasia, *Brain and Language* **29**, 48–67

Ryalls, J. H. and Lieberman, P. (1982) Fundamental frequency and vowel perception, *Journal of the Acoustical Society of America* **72**, 1631–4

Sachs, J., Lieberman, P. and Erickson, D. (1972) Anatomical and cultural determinants of male and female speech. *In Language attitudes: Current trends and prospects*. Washington, DC: Georgetown University Series in Language and Linguistics

Sandner, G. W. (1981) Communication with a three-month-old baby. *In Proceedings of Thirteenth Annual Child Language Research Forum*. Stanford, Calif: Child Language Project, Stanford University

Sawashima, M. (1974) Laryngeal research in experimental phonetics. *In* T. Sebeok (ed.), *Current trends in linguistics, Vol. 12*. The Hague: Mouton

Sawashima, M. and Hirose, H. (1968) New laryngoscopic technique by use of fiberoptics, *Journal of the Acoustical Society of America* **43**, 168–9

Sawashima, M. and Miyazaki, S. (1973) Glottal opening for Japanese voiceless consonants, *Annual Bulletin of the Research Institute of Logopedics and Phoniatrics, University of Tokyo* **7**, 1–9

Scherer, K. R. (1981) Speech and emotional states. *In* J. K. Darby (ed.) *Speech evaluation in psychiatry*. New York: Grune and Stratton

Searle, C. L., Jacobson, J. Z. and Rayment, S. G. (1979) Phoneme recognition based on human audition, *Journal of the Acoustical Society of America* **65**, 799–809

Shadle, C. H. (1985) Intrinsic fundamental frequency of vowels in sentence context, *Journal of the Acoustical Society of America* **78**, 1562–7

Shankweiler, D. and Studdert-Kennedy, M. (1967) Identification of consonants and vowels presented to left and right ears, *Quarterly Journal of Experimental Psychology* **19**, 59–63

Sharf, B. (1970) Critical bands. *In* J. V. Tobias (ed.) *Foundations of modern auditory theory, Vol. 1*. New York: Academic Press

Shewan, C. M., Leeper, H. A. and Booth, J. C. (1984) An analysis of voice onset time (VOT) in aphasic and normal subjects. *In* J. Rosenbek, M. McNeil and A. Aronson (eds.), *Apraxia of speech: Physiology, acoustics, linguistics, management*. San Diego: College-Hill Press

Shinn, P. and Blumstein, S. E. (1983) Phonetic disintegration in aphasia: Acoustic analysis of spectral characteristics for place of articulation, *Brain and Language* **20**, 90–114

Shipp, T. and McGlone, R. E. (1971) Laryngeal dynamics associated with vocal frequency change, *Journal of Speech and Hearing Research* **14**, 761–8

Shipp, T., Doherty, E. T. and Morrisey, T. (1979) Predicting vocal frequency from selected physiologic measures, *Journal of the Acoustical Society of America* **66**, 678–84

Simada, Z. and Hirose, H. (1970) The function of the laryngeal muscles in respect to the word accent distinction, *Annual Bulletin of the Research Institute of Logopedics and Phoniatrics, University of Tokyo* **4**, 27–40

Snow, C. E. (1977) Mother's speech research: from input to interaction. *In* C. E. Snow and C. A. Ferguson (eds.), *Talking to children: language input and acquisition.* Cambridge: Cambridge University Press

Soli, S. (1981) Second formants in fricatives: Acoustic consequences of fricative-vowel coarticulation, *Journal of the Acoustical Society of America* **70**, 976–84

Stetson, R. H. (1951) *Motor phonetics,* 2nd ed. Amsterdam: North Holland

Stevens, K. N. (1972a) Airflow and turbulence noise for fricative and stop consonants: Static considerations, *Journal of the Acoustical Society of America* **50**, 1182–92

Stevens, K. N. (1972b) Quantal nature of speech. *In* E. E. David Jr and P. B. Denes (eds.), *Human communication: A unified view.* New York: McGraw-Hill

Stevens, K. N. (1985) Evidence for the role of acoustic boundaries in the perception of speech sounds *In* V. A. Fromkin (ed.), *Phonetic linguistics: Essays in honor of Peter Ladefoged.* New York: Academic Press

Stevens, K. N. and Blumstein, S. E. (1979) Invariant cues for place of articulation in stop consonants, *Journal of the Acoustical Society of America* **64**, 1358–68

Stevens, K. N. and Blumstein, S. E. (1981) The search for invariant acoustic correlates of phonetic features. *In* P. D. Eimas and J. L. Miller (eds.), *Perspectives on the study of speech.* New Jersey: Erlbaum

Stevens, K. N. and House, A. S. (1955) Development of a quantitative description of vowel articulation, *Journal of the Acoustical Society of America* **27**, 484–93

Stevens, K. N. and House, A. S. (1961) An acoustical theory of vowel production and some of its implications, *Journal of Speech and Hearing Research* **4**, 303–20

Stevens, K. N. and Klatt, D. H. (1974) Role of formant transitions in the voiced–voiceless distinction of stops, *Journal of the Acoustical Society of America* **55**, 653–9

Stevens, K. N., Bastide, R. P. and Smith, C. P. (1955) Electrical synthesizer of continuous speech, *Journal of the Acoustical Society of America* **25**, 207

Stevens, K. N., Kasouski, S. and Fant, C. G. M. (1953) An electrical analog of the vocal tract, *Journal of the Acoustical Society of America* **25**, 734–42

Stevens, K. N., Liberman, A. M. and Studdert-Kennedy, M. (1969) Cross-language study of vowel perception, *Language and Speech* **12**, 1–23

Stevens, S. S. and Davis, H. (1938) *Hearing.* New York: John Wiley and Sons

Strange, W., Verbrugge, R. R., Shankweiler, D. P. and Edman, T. R. (1976) Consonantal environment specifies vowel identify, *Journal of the Acoustical Society of America* **60**, 213–24

Strevens, P. (1960) Spectra of fricative noise in human speech, *Language Speech* **3**, 32–49

Stuart, R. R. (1958) *The anatomy of the bullfrog.* Denoyer-Geppert

Summerfield, A. Q. (1975) How a full account of segmental perception depends on prosody and vice versa. *In* A. Cohen and S. G. Nooteboom (eds.), *Structure and process in speech perception.* New York: Springer-Verlag

Timcke, R., Von Leden, H. and Moore, P. (1958) Laryngeal vibrations: Measurements of the glottic wave, *AMA Archives of Otolaryngology* **68**, 1–19

Tosi, O., Oyer, H., Lashbrook, W., Pedrey, J., Nichol, J. and Nash, E. (1972) Experiment on voice identification, *Journal of the Acoustical Society of America* **51**, 2030–43

Trubetzkoy, N. S. (1939) Grundzuge der phonologie, *Travaux du Cercle Linguistique de Prague* **7**, Prague

Truby, H. M., Bosma, J. F. and Lind, J. (1965) *Newborn infant cry.* Almquist and Wiksell

Tseng, C. Y. (1981) An acoustic study of tones in Mandarin. Unpublished Ph.D. thesis, Brown University

Tuller, B. (1984) On categorizing speech errors, *Neuropsychologia* **22**, 547–58

Tuller, B. and Kelso, J. A. Scott (1984) The timing of articulatory gestures: Evidence for relational invariants, *Journal of the Acoustical Society of America* **76**, 1030–6

Umeda, N. (1975) Vowel duration in American English, *Journal of the Acoustical Society of America*, **58**, 434–45

Umeda, N. (1982) F_0 declination is situation dependent, *Journal of Phonetics* **10**, 279–90

Van den Berg, J. (1958) Myoelastic-aerodynamic theory of voice production. *Journal of Speech and Hearing Research* **1**, 227–44

Van den Berg, J. (1960) Vocal ligaments versus registers, *Current Problems in Phoniatrics and Logopedics* **1**, 19–34

Van den Berg, J. (1962) Modern research in experimental phoniatrics, *Folia Phoniatrica* **14**, 81–149

Vanderslice, R. and Ladefoged, P. (1972) Binary suprasegmental features and transformational word-accentuation rules, *Language* **48**, 819–38

von Kempelin, W. R. 1791. *Mechanismum der menschlichen Sprache nebst der Beschreibung seiner sprechenden Maschine*. J. B. Degen

Watkin, K. and Fromm, D. (1984) Labial coordination in children: Preliminary considerations, *Journal of the Acoustical Society of America* **75**, 629–32

Werker, J. F., Gilbert, J. H. V., Humphrey, K. and Tees, R. C. (1981) Developmental aspects of cross-language speech perception, *Child Development* **52**, 349–55

Werker, J. F. and Tees, R. C. (1984) Cross-language speech perception: Evidence for perceptual reorganization during the first year of life, *Infant Behavior and Development* **7**, 49–63

Wernicke, C. (1874) *Der aphasische Symptomenkomplex*. Breslau: Cohn and Weigert

Wollberg, Z. and Newman, J. D. (1972) Auditory cortex of squirrel monkey: Response patterns of single cells to species-specific vocalizations, *Science* **175**, 212–14

Wood, C. C., Goff, W. R. and Day, R. S. (1971) Auditory evoked potentials during speech perception, *Science* **173**, 1248—51

Yanagihara, N. and Hyde, C. (1966) An aerodynamic study of the articulatory mechanism in the production of bilabial stop consonants, *Studia Phonetica* **4**, 70–80

Yeni-Komshian, G. and Soli, S. (1981) Recognition of vowels from information in fricatives: Perceptual evidence of fricative-vowel coarticulation, *Journal of the Acoustical Society of America* **70**, 966–75

Zemlin, W. R. (1968) *Speech and hearing science, anatomy and physiology*. Englewood Cliffs, NJ: Prentice Hall

Ziegler, W. and Von Cramon, D. (1985) Anticipatory co-articulation in a patient with apraxia of speech, *Brain and Language* **26**, 117–30

Zwicker, E. (1961) Subdivision of the audible frequency range into critical bands (Frequenzgruppen), *Journal of the Acoustical Society of America* **33**, 248

Zwislocki, J. (1965) Analysis of some auditory characteristics. *In* R. D. Luce, R. R. Bush, and E. Galanter (eds.) *Handbook of mathematic psychology, Vol. 3*, New York: Wiley

Index